W0080627

Haematological Disorders in Pregnancy

Haematological Disorders in Pregnancy

Editors

Komal N Chavan
MD, DNB, MNAMS, FCPS, DGO, FICOG, Diploma in Reproductive Medicine (UKSH, Germany)

Chairperson, FOGSI Medical Disorders in Pregnancy Committee (2019–2021)
Medical Director–Consultant, Chavan Maternity and Nursing Home, Mumbai
Honorary Assistant Professor, HBT Medical College and
Dr RN Cooper Municipal General Hospital, Mumbai

Niranjan Chavan
MD, FICOG, FCPS, DGO, DFP, MICOG, DICOG, Diploma in Endoscopy (USA)

Professor and Unit Chief
Lokmanya Tilak Municipal General Hospital and Medical College, Mumbai
National Coordinator, FOGSI Medical Disorders in Pregnancy Committee (2019–2021)
Secretary, MOGS (2019–2020); Member, Oncology Committee AOFOG (2013–2015)
Chairperson, FOGSI Oncology and TT Committee (2012–2014)
Course Coordinator, Advanced Minimal Access Gynaec. Surgery
Lokmanya Tilak Municipal General Hospital and Medical College, Mumbai
Medical Director–Consultant, Chavan Maternity and Nursing Home, Mumbai

Co-editors

Dinesh Wade
Vibhusha Rohidas

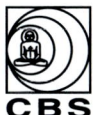

CBS Publishers & Distributors Pvt Ltd

New Delhi • Bengaluru • Chennai • Kochi • Kolkata • Mumbai
Bhopal • Bhubaneswar • Hyderabad • Jharkhand • Nagpur • Patna • Pune
Uttarakhand • Dhaka (Bangladesh) • Kathmandu (Nepal)

Disclaimer

Science and technology are constantly changing fields. New research and experience broaden the scope of information and knowledge. The editors have tried their best in giving information available to them while preparing the material for this book. Although, all efforts have been made to ensure optimum accuracy of the material, yet it is quite possible some errors might have been left uncorrected. The publisher, the editors and the printer will not be held responsible for any inadvertent errors, or inaccuracies.

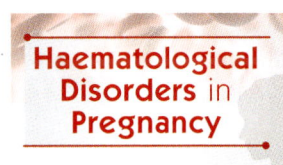

Haematological Disorders in Pregnancy

ISBN: 978-93-89017-62-5

Copyright © Editors and Publisher

First Edition: 2020

All rights reserved. No part of this book may be reproduced or transmitted in any form or by any means, electronic or mechanical, including photocopying, recording, or any information storage and retrieval system without permission, in writing, from the editors and the publisher.

Published by Satish Kumar Jain and produced by Varun Jain for

CBS Publishers & Distributors Pvt Ltd
4819/XI Prahlad Street, 24 Ansari Road, Daryaganj, New Delhi 110 002, India.
Ph: 23289259, 23266861, 23266867   Website: www.cbspd.com
Fax: 011-23243014   e-mail: delhi@cbspd.com; cbspubs@airtelmail.in.
Corporate Office: 204 FIE, Industrial Area, Patparganj, Delhi 110 092

Ph: 4934 4934   Fax: 4934 4935   e-mail: publishing@cbspd.com; publicity@cbspd.com

Branches

- **Bengaluru:** Seema House 2975, 17th Cross, K.R. Road,
  Banasankari 2nd Stage, Bengaluru 560 070, Karnataka
  Ph: +91-80-26771678/79   Fax: +91-80-26771680   e-mail: bangalore@cbspd.com
- **Chennai:** 7, Subbaraya Street, Shenoy Nagar, Chennai 600 030, Tamil Nadu
  Ph: +91-44-26680620, 26681266   Fax: +91-44-42032115   e-mail: chennai@cbspd.com
- **Kochi:** 68/1534, 35, 36, Power House Road, Opp. KSEB, Kochi 682018, Kerala
  Ph: +91-484-4059061-65   Fax: +91-484-4059065   e-mail: kochi@cbspd.com
- **Kolkata:** 6/B, Ground Floor, Rameswar Shaw Road, Kolkata-700 014, West Bengal
  Ph: +91-33-22891126, 22891127, 22891128   e-mail: kolkata@cbspd.com
- **Mumbai:** 83-C, Dr E Moses Road, Worli, Mumbai-400018, Maharashtra
  Ph: +91-22-24902340/41   Fax: +91-22-24902342   e-mail: mumbai@cbspd.com

Representatives

- **Bhopal**   0-8319310552 • **Bhubaneswar**   0-9911037372 • **Hyderabad** 0-9885175004 • **Jharkhand**   0-9811541605
- **Nagpur**   0-9421945513 • **Patna**   0-9334159340 • **Pune**   0-9623451994 • **Uttarakhand** 0-9716462459
- **Dhaka (Bangladesh)** 01912-003485 • **Kathmandu (Nepal)** 977-9818742655

Printed at Nutech Print Services, Faridabad, Haryana, India

Foreword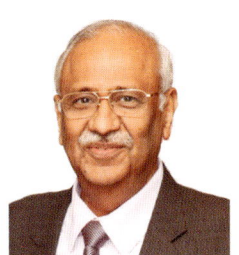

Dear FOGSIans

It gives me immense pleasure to write a foreword to the monograph *Haematological Disorders in Pregnancy* authored and edited by Dr Komal N Chavan, Chairperson, FOGSI Medical Disorders in Pregnancy Committee, and Dr Niranjan Chavan, Professor and Unit Chief, Lokmanya Tilak Municipal General Hospital and Medical College, Mumbai.

The monograph covers basic haematology and progresses to haematological disorders in pregnancy, haemoglobinopathies, and oncology. It has lucid presentation and each chapter has numerous colour pictures, tables and refer the latest guidelines and journals which will be a desktop ready-reckoner for obstetricians in their day-to- day practice.

It encompasses preventive, diagnostic and treatment modalities of various types of anaemias and haemoglobinopathies which will help to reduce the maternal morbidity and mortality of India.

Use of newer parenteral iron preparations such a ferric carboxymaltose (FCM) will be beneficial not only to patients with anaemia during postpartum period but now can be given safely in antenatal period.

This will be the first monograph in the series of 12 monographs and I wish both Dr Komal Chavan and Dr Niranjan Chavan, all the best for their future endeavours in their goals to reduce anaemia in pregnancy and social contributions in academic organisations.

With warm personal regards

MB Agarwal MD, MNAMS
Professor and Head, Department of Haematology
Bombay Hospital Institute of Medical Sciences
Mumbai

● Foreword

I am grateful to Dr Komal N Chavan, Chairperson of the FOGSI Committee on Medical Disorders Compilcating Pregnancy, for inviting me to write a foreword to this monograph entitled *Haematological Disorders in Pregnancy*.

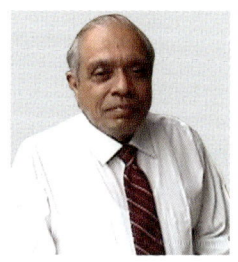

Anaemia takes the prime position amongst the various medical disorders in pregnancy. It is widely prevalent in India. It is an important factor contributing to adverse obstetric outcomes in pregnancy. It is estimated that anaemia contributes to around 20% of all maternal deaths in our country.

The ICMR reported the prevalence of mild, moderate and severe anaemia to be 13%, 57% and 12% (overall >80%) in a pan India study, thus establishing it as the most common medical disorder complicating pregnancy calling for urgent attention.

Nutritional deficiencies account for the majority of cases. Iron deficiency anaemia which leads the causes is easily detectable and correctable. Folate deficiency accounts for 0.5–3% of the population and is amenable to therapy.

Worm infestations are prevalent amongst the farming community and are treatable. However, haemoglobinopathies affect certain communities, if left unrecognised— these can lead to adverse outcomes.

Haemophilias and thrombophilias though uncommon, need counselling.

Antenatal care is of prime importance in detecting and treating haematological disorders during pregnancy. Women with rare haematological problems should be referred to higher centres for special care.

This monograph aims at drawing attention to the role of haematological disorders complicating pregnancy and the importance of their recognition and management. My congratulations to Dr Komal N Chavan for highlighting this important area of pregnancy care to promote safe motherhood.

Shirish N Daftary

Past President, FOGSI

Foreword

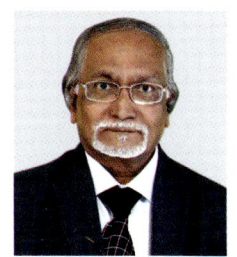

The horizon of knowledge in obstetrics and gynaecology keeps widening day by day. The clinicians and the postgraduate students must be aware of the latest in the field. Timely execution of updated knowledge can save life during pregnancy. Busy practitioners and residents do not have adequate time to update themselves with latest in the field.

Dr Komal N Chavan, Chairperson of FOGSI Committee on Medical Disorders in Pregnancy, has come out with this monograph *Haematological Disorders in Pregnancy*. This monograph covers a wide range of topics starting with basic morphology of RBCs and haem molecule, progressing to completely covering various types of anaemias, platelet disorders, DIC during pregnancy.

I am confident that the information provided in this monograph will tremendously help FOGSI members and postgraduate students in efficiently managing wide range of haematological disorders in pregnancy.

I congratulate editors Dr Komal N Chavan and Dr Niranjan Chavan for selection of this topic and efforts put in.

I am sure after reading and understanding contents of this monograph every FOGSI member and postgraduate student would be looking forward to release of such monographs every three months by Dr Komal N Chavan and Dr Niranjan Chavan.

PK Shah

Professer and Unit Head, Department of Obs & Gyn.
LTMG Hospital, Mumbai (1995–2008)
Professer and Unit Head, Department of Obs & Gyn.
Seth GS Medical College and KEM Hospital, Mumbai (2008–2016)
Past President, FOGSI, IAGE, IFUMB, MOGS, AFTT
Past Dean, Indian College of Medical Ultrasound (2014–2016)
Past Editor, *Obs & Gyn. Today Journal*
Member, USG Committee, AOFOG (2000–2016)
Member, Safe Motherhood Committee, FIGO (2013–2018)
Chairman, Imaging Science Committee, SAFOG (2017–2019)
Past Chairman, Imaging Science Committee, FOGSI (2001–2005)

Message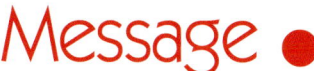

Dear readers

Greetings from the FOGSI President and her team!

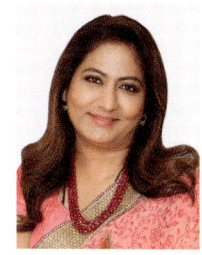

Treating medical disorders during pregnancy is a challenge for all of us obstetricians as we are responsible for both the patient and the baby. Ensuring the optimum care at every stage for haematological conditions, which are among the most challenging issues faced by us, is very important.

This book aims to present at a glance the various haematological disorders encountered in clinical practice and to provide the current evidence on the treatment protocols for these issues.

Life's challenges are not supposed to paralyse you. They are supposed to help you discover who you are.
—Bernice Johnson Reagan

I congratulate the authors, editors and the Chairperson of the Medical Disorders in Pregnancy Committee, Dr Komal N Chavan, for their efforts in bringing this unique book to you. I have no doubt that it will go a long way towards answering many of your doubts and will help you tackle haematological disorders, the obstetric and medical crises that present in day-to-day practice.

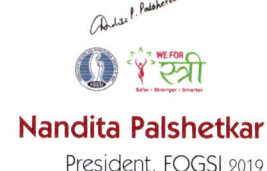

Nandita Palshetkar
President, FOGSI 2019

Preface

It gives me immense pleasure to present to you the first monograph *Haematological Disorders in Pregnancy,* one of the series of 12 monographs planned. Anaemia is the leading cause of maternal mortality in India and Ministry of Health has launched Anaemia *Mukt Bharat* Mission—target 2022. As a Chairperson of FOGSI Medical Disorders in Pregnancy Committee, my main focus is on prevention, early diagnosis, and management of haematological disorders in pregnancy.

We gynaecologists are the first ones to detect and diagnose anaemia in our pregnant patients. This book contains the physiology and morphology of RBC, physiological changes in pregnancy, management of anaemia and other haematological disorders in pregnancy. It is a handy book with colour diagrams, flowcharts and it will be a 'must read' for all the aspiring and practising gynaecologists.

I would also express my deep gratitude to Dr MB Agarwal, Dr Shirish Daftary and Dr PK Shah for giving foreword to this monograph. Message by Dr Nandita Palshetkar, President, FOGSI, is very motivating and inspiring us to do not only our academic but social responsibility with the theme

We For Stree — Stronger, Safer, Smarter.

I would like to thank Dr Niranjan Chavan, my husband, who has always been kind and supportive in my academic endeavours and edited this book with me along with my co-editors Dr Dinesh Wade and Dr Vibhusha Rohidas who burnt the midnight oil. I would also like to thank Mr Ramesh Krishnamachari of CBS Publishers & Distributors who was very efficient, cooperative in getting this monograph printed at the earliest.

The journey from installation as a chairperson on 9th January 2019 at the AICOG 2019, Bengaluru, till the release of this first monograph at North Zone Yuva FOGSI on 2nd February 2019, has been wonderful with my team who have made my dream come true.

Happy reading to you all !!

With Warm Regards

Komal N Chavan
Chairperson
FOGSI Medical Disorders in
Pregnancy Committee (2019–2021)

Contents

Abbreviations

WHO	World Health Organisation
ID	Iron Deficiency
RBC's	Red Blood Cells
PHSC	Pluripotent Haemopoietic Stem Cells
LSC	Lymphoid Stem Cells
NK	Natural Killer
CFU-E	Colony Forming Unit-Erythrocytes
CFU-GM	Colony Forming Unit-Granulocytes/Monocytes
CFU-M	Colony Forming Unit-Megakaryocytes
Hb	Haemoglobin
CO	Carbon Monoxide
NADH	Nicotinamide Adenine Dinucleotide
NADPH	Nicotinamide Adenine Dinucleotide Phosphate
ALA	Aminolevulinic Acid
IDA	Iron Deficiency Anaemia
FCM	Ferric Carboxymaltose
HR-QOL	Health-Related Quality-of-Life
rhEPO	Recombinant Erythropoietin
HIV	Human Immune Virus
DIC	Disseminated Intravascular Coagulation
FDP	Fibrin Degradation Product
TT	Thrombin Time
PT	Prothrombin Time
INR	International Normalised Ratio
PTT	Partial Thromboplastin Time
ISTH	International Society on Thrombosis and Haemostasis
JMHW	Japanese Ministry of Health and Welfare
JAAM	Japanese Association for Acute Medicine
MCV	Mean Cell Volume

MCH   Mean Corpuscular Haemoglobin

MCHC   Mean Corpuscular Haemoglobin Concentration

PCR   Polymerase Chain Reaction

ITP   Idiopathic Thrombocytopenic Purpura

IVIG   Intravenous Immune Globin

ASH   American Society of Haematology

BCSH   British Society of Haematology

TTP   Thrombotic Thrombocytopenic Purpura

HUS   Haemolytic Uremic Syndrome

AST   Aspartate Transaminase

ALT   Alanine Transaminase

Introduction

Worldwide, anaemia affects over 2 billion people and the World Health Organization (WHO) has esimated that half of these are due to iron deficiency. Iron deficiency is not only the most prevalent but also the most neglected nutrient deficiency in the world, mostly among pregnant women and children in under developed countries. Currently, over fourty million pregnant ladies suffer from iron deficiency (ID) and its consequences in developing countries.

Iron deficiency is the most common cause of anaemia in pregnancy. Iron deficiency anaemia accounts for 75–95% of cases of anaemia in pregnancy. Iron deficiency anaemia, the late manifestation of chronic iron deficiency, is thought to be the most common nutrient deficiency among pregnant women. Studies conducted on pregnant women in African countries, China, India, and Mexico from 1996 to 2008 indicated that between 43% and 73% of the women were iron deficient (usually diagnosed as a low-ferritin concentration); out of these, 7–33% had IDA.

Among pregnant women, IDA has been associated with increased risks of low birth weight, prematurity, and maternal morbidity. UNICEF has reported deaths of an estimated 50,000 young women per year globally in pregnancy and childbirth due to severe iron deficiency anemia. The high frequency of iron deficiency anaemia within the developing countries has substantial health and economic cost implications. An analysis of 10 developing countries reported $0.32 per head or 0.57% of gross domestic product as a median value of physical productivity loss per year resulting from iron deficiency.

Red Blood Cells

Red blood cells (RBCs) are the non-nucleated elements in the blood and also known as erythrocytes (erythros = red) (Fig. 2.1). Red colour of the red blood cell is due to the colouring pigment called haemoglobin. RBCs play a significant role in transport of respiratory gases. RBCs are larger in number as compared to the other two blood cells, like white blood cells and platelets.

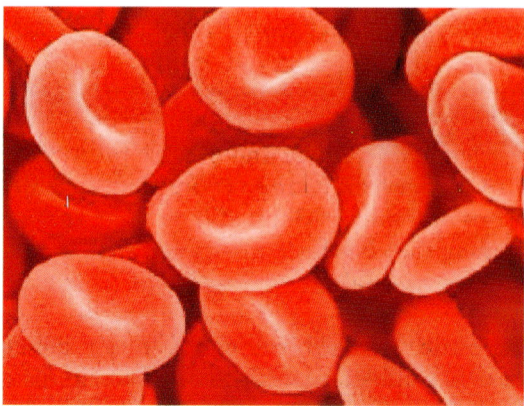

Fig. 2.1: Normal structure of RBC

NORMAL VALUE

RBC count varies between 4 and 5.5 million/cmm of blood.
Adult males—5 million/cmm
Adult females—4.5 million/cmm.

MORPHOLOGY OF RED BLOOD CELLS

Normal Shape

The RBCs are disk-shaped and biconcave (dumbbell-shaped). Due biconcave contour of RBCs has some mechanical and functional advantages. Central portion is thinner and periphery is thicker (Fig. 2.2)

Advantages of biconcave shape of RBCs

1. Large surface area is provided for absorption or removal of different substances.
2. Biconcave shape helps in equal and rapid diffusion of oxygen and other substances into the interior of the cell.

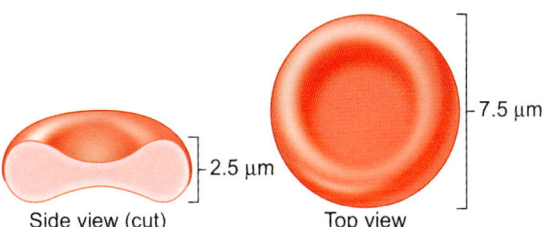

Fig. 2.2: Shape of RBC

3. Minimal tension is offered to the membrane when the volume of cell changes.
4. Due biconcave shape, while passing through small capillaries, RBCs squeeze through the capillaries very easily without damage to its structure.

Normal Size

Diameter: 7.2 (6.9 to 7.4).

Thickness: At the periphery it is thicker with 2.2. At the center it is thinner with 1. This difference in thickness is due to the biconcave shape.

Surface area: 120 sq.

Volume: 85 to 90 cu.

Normal Structure

Red blood cells are non-nucleated. Due to the absence of nucleus in human RBC, the DNA is also absent. Other organelles like mitochondria and Golgi apparatus also are absent in RBC. Due to absence of mitochondria, the energy is produced from glycolytic process. Red cell lacks insulin receptor and so the glucose uptake by this cell is not controlled by insulin. It has a special type of cytoskeleton, which is made up of actin and spectrin. Both of these proteins are anchored to transmembrane proteins by means of another protein named ankyrin. Hereditary spherocytosis occurs due to absence of spectrin. And hence, the cell is deformed, losses its biconcave shape and it becomes globular (spherocytic). The spherocyte is very fragile and can easily ruptured (hemolysed) in hypotonic solutions.

PROPERTIES OF RED BLOOD CELLS

Rouleaux Formation

When blood is taken out of the blood vessel, the RBCs pile up one above another like the pile of coins. This property of the RBCs is named rouleaux (pleural = rouleau) formation (Fig. 2.3). It is accelerated by plasma proteins globulin and fibrinogen.

Specific Gravity

Specific gravity of RBC is 1.092 to 1.101.

Packed Cell Volume

Packed cell volume (PCV) is the proportion of blood occupied by RBCs expressed in percentage. It is also called haematocrit value. It is 45% of the blood and the plasma volume is 55%.

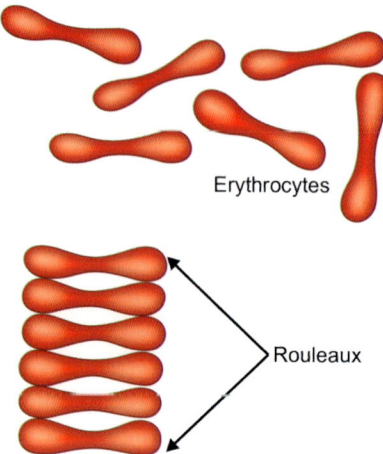

Fig. 2.3: Rouleaux formation

Suspension Stability

During circulation, the RBCs remain suspended uniformly in the blood. This property of the RBCs is called the suspension stability.

Lifespan of Red Blood Cells

Average lifespan of RBC is about 120 days. After the lifetime the senile (old) RBCs are destroyed in reticuloendothelial system.

Determination of Lifespan of Red Blood Cells

Lifespan of the RBC is determined by radioisotope method. RBCs are tagged with radioactive substances like radioactive iron or radioactive chromium. Life of RBC is determined by studying the rate of loss of radioactive cells from circulation.

Fate of Red Blood Cells

When the cells die (120 days), the cell membrane becomes more fragile. Diameter of the capillaries is less or equal to that of RBC. Younger RBCs can pass through the capillaries easily. However, due to the delicate nature, the older cells are destroyed while trying to squeeze through the capillaries. The destruction happens primarily in the capillaries of red pulp of spleen as the diameter of splenic capillaries is extremely small. So, the spleen is called 'graveyard of RBCs'. Destroyed RBCs are fragmented and haemoglobin is released from the fragmented parts. Haemoglobin is immediately phagocytised by macrophages of the body, particularly the macrophages present in liver (Kupffer cells), spleen and bone marrow.

Haemoglobin is degraded into iron, globin and porphyrin. Iron combines with apoferritin to form ferritin, which is stored in the body and reused later. Globin enters the protein depot for later use. Porphyrin is degraded into bilirubin, which is excreted by liver through bile. Daily 10% RBCs, which are senile, are destroyed in normal young healthy adults. It causes release of about 0.6 g/dL of haemoglobin into the plasma. From this 0.9 to 1.5 mg/dL bilirubin is formed.

Functions of Red Blood Cells

Major function of RBCs is the transport of respiratory gases. Following are the functions of:

RBCs

Transport of oxygen from the lungs to the tissues

Haemoglobin in RBC combines with oxygen to form oxyhaemoglobin. About 97% of oxygen is transported in blood in the form of oxyhaemoglobin.

Transport of carbon dioxide from the tissues to the lungs

Haemoglobin combines with carbon dioxide and form carbhaemoglobin. About 30% of carbon dioxide is transportedin this form. RBCs contain a large amount of the carbonic anhydrase. This enzyme is necessary for the formation of bicarbonate from water and carbondioxide. Thus, it helps to transport carbon dioxide in the form of bicarbonate from tissues to lungs. About 63% of carbon dioxide is transported in this form.

Buffering action in blood

Haemoglobin functions as a good buffer. By this action, it regulates the hydrogen ion concentration and thereby plays a role in the maintenance of acid–base balance.

In blood group determination

RBCs carry the blood group antigens like A antigen, B antigen and Rh factor. This helps in determination of blood group and enables to prevent reactions due to incompatible blood transfusion.

VARIATIONS IN NUMBER OF RED BLOOD CELLS

Physiological Variations

Increase in RBC Count

Increase in the RBC count is known as polycythemia. It occurs in both physiological and pathological conditions. When it occurs in physiological conditions it is called physiological polycythemia. The increase in number during this condition is marginal and temporary. It occurs in the following conditions:

Age: At birth, the RBC count is 8 to 10 million/cmm of blood. The count decreases within 10 days after birth due to destruction of RBCs causing physiological jaundice in some newborn babies. However, in infants and growing children, the cell count is more than the value in adults.

Sex: Before puberty and after menopause in females the RBC count is similar to that in males. During reproductive period of females, the count is less than that of males (4.5 million/cmm).

High altitude: Inhabitants of mountains (above 10,000 feet from mean sea level) have an increased RBC count of more than 7 million/cmm. It is due to hypoxia (decreased oxygen supply to tissues) in high altitude. Hypoxia stimulates kidney to secrete a hormone called erythropoietin. The erythropoietin in turn stimulates the bone marrow to produce more RBCs.

Muscular exercise: There is a temporary increase in RBC count after exercise. It is because of mild hypoxia and contraction of spleen. Spleen stores RBCs. Hypoxia increases the sympathetic activity leading to secretion of adrenaline from adrenal medulla. Adrenaline contracts spleen and RBCs are released into blood.

Emotional conditions: RBC count increases through the emotional conditions like anxiety. It is as a result of increase in the sympathetic activity as in the case of muscular exercise.

Increased environmental temperature: Increase in atmospheric temperature will increases RBC count. Generally increased temperature increases all the activities in the body as well as production of RBCs.

After meals: There is a small increase in the RBC count when taking meals. It is because of need for more oxygen for metabolic activities.

Decrease in RBC Count

Decrease in RBC Count Occurs in the following Physiological Conditions

High barometric pressures: At high barometric pressures as in deep sea, when the oxygen tension of blood is higher, the RBC count decreases.

During sleep: RBC count decreases slightly throughout sleep and immediately after getting up from sleep. Generally all the activities of the body are decreased during sleep including production of RBCs.

Pregnancy: In pregnancy, the RBC count decreases. It is because of increase in ECF volume. Increase in ECF volume, increases the plasma volume also resulting in haemodilution. So, there is a relative reduction in the RBC count.

Pathological Variations

Pathological Polycythaemia

Pathological polycythaemia is the abnormal increase in the RBC count. Red cell count increases above 7 million/cmm of the blood. Polycythaemia is of two types, the primary polycythaemia and secondary polycythaemia.

Primary Polycythaemia—Polycythaemia Vera

Primary polycythaemia is otherwise known as polycythaemia vera. It is a disease characterised by persistent increase in RBC count above 14 million/cmm of blood. This is always associated with increased white blood cell count above 24,000/cmm of blood. Polycythaemia vera occurs in myeloproliferative disorders like malignancy of red bone marrow.

Secondary Polycythaemia

This is secondary to a number of the pathological conditions (diseases) such as:
1. Respiratory disorders like emphysema.
2. Congenital heart disease.
3. Ayerza's disease (condition associated with hypertrophy of right ventricle and obstruction of blood flow to lungs).
4. Chronic carbon monoxide poisoning.

5. Poisoning by chemicals like phosphorus and arsenic.
6. Repeated mild haemorrhages.

All these conditions lead to hypoxia which stimulates the release of erythropoietin. Erythropoietin stimulates the bone marrow resulting in increased RBC count.

Anaemia

Abnormal decrease in RBC count is called anaemia.

Variations in Size of Red Blood Cells

Under physiological conditions, the size of RBCs in venous blood is slightly larger than those in arterial blood. In pathological conditions, the variations in size of RBCs are:
1. Microcytes (smaller cells).
2. Macrocytes (larger cells).
3. Anisocytes (cells with different sizes).

MICROCYTES

Microcytes are present in:

i. Iron deficiency anaemia.
ii. Prolonged forced breathing.
iii. Increased osmotic pressure in blood.

MACROCYTES

Macrocytes are present in:

i. Megaloblastic anaemia.
ii. Decreased osmotic pressure in blood.

ANISOCYTES

Anisocytes occurs in pernicious anaemia.

Variations in Shape of Red Blood Cells

Shape of RBCs is altered in many conditions including different types of anaemia.

1. Crenation: Shrinkage as in hypertonic conditions.
2. Spherocytosis: Globular form as in hypotonic conditions.
3. Elliptocytosis: Elliptical shape as in certain types of anaemia.
4. Sickle cell: Crescentic shape as in sickle cell anaemia.
5. Poikilocytosis: Unusual shapes due to deformed cell membrane. The shape will be of flask, hammer or any other unusual shape.

VARIATIONS IN STRUCTURE OF RED BLOOD CELLS

Punctate Basophilism

Striated appearance of RBCs by the presence of dots of basophilic materials (porphyrin) is called punctuate basophilism (Fig. 2.4). It occurs in conditions like lead poisoning.

Ring in Red Blood Cells

Ring or twisted strands of basophilic material appear in the periphery of the RBCs. This is also called the Goblet ring. This appears in the RBCs in certain types of anaemia.

Howell-Jolly Bodies

In certain types of anaemia, some nuclear fragments are present in the ectoplasm of the RBCs. These nuclear fragments are called Howell-Jolly bodies (Figs 2.5 and 2.6).

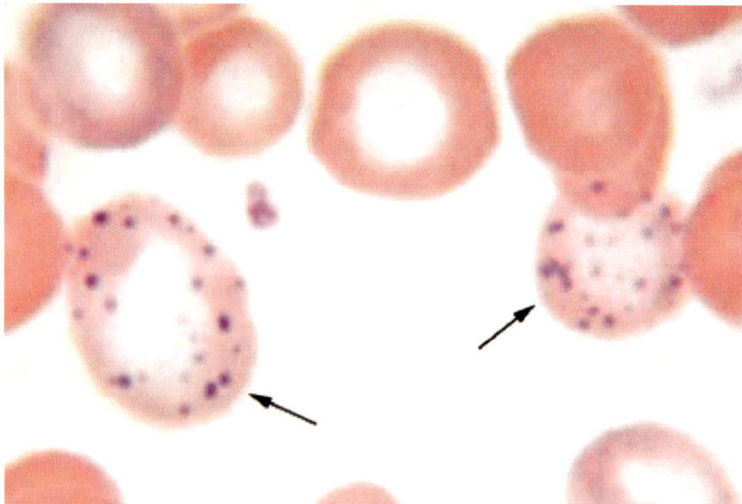

Fig. 2.4: Punctuate basophilia

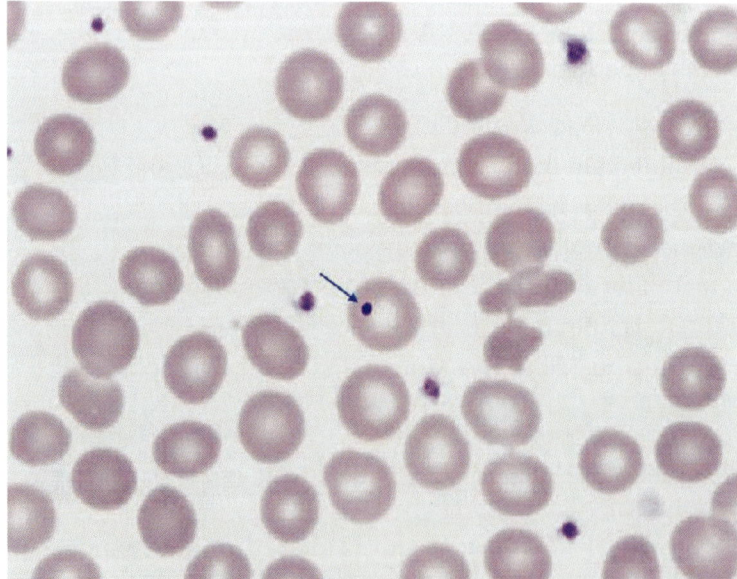

Fig. 2.5: Howell-Jolly bodies

Abnormal RBC morphology	Cartoon image	May be associated with
Microcytic RBC	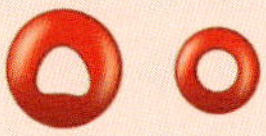	Pyridoxine deficiency Thalassaemia Iron deficiency anaemia Chronic disease anaemia (sometimes) Sideroblastic anaemia (sometimes)
Macrocytic RBC	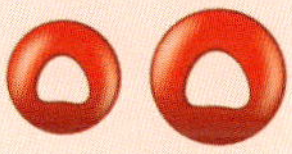	Vitamin B_{12} or follate deficiency Liver disease MDS Chemotherapy (e.g. methotrexate)
Spurr cell RBC (acanthocyte)	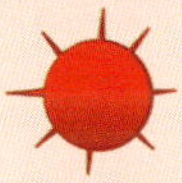	Abetalipoproteinemia Liver disease McLeod blood group phenotype Post-splenectomy, etc.
Burr cell RBC (echinocyte)	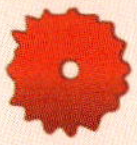	Artitact Anaemia Liver disease, etc.
Schistocyte	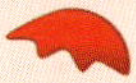	Microangiopathic Haemolytic anaemia Mechanical valve induced, etc.
Bite cell RBC	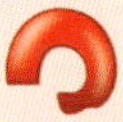	GSPD deficiency Unstable haemoglobin disorders Oxidative drugs
Elliptocyte	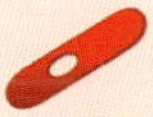	Hereditary elliptocytosis Severe iron deficiency anaemia
Spherocyte	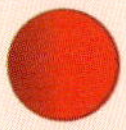	Hereditary sphenocytosis Autoimmune haemolytic anaemia
Stomatocyte	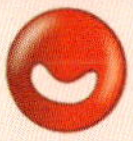	Hereditary stomatocytosis Liver disease
Target cell RBC	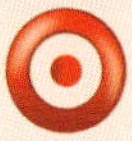	Thalassaemia Haemoglobinopathies Postsplenectomy Liver disease Artitact
Sickle cell RBC	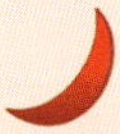	Haemoglobin SS disease Haemoglobin SC disease Haemoglobin SD disease S beta thalassaemia
Tear drop	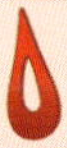	Myelofibrosis Underlying narrow process filltrate, etc.
Haemoglobin C crystals	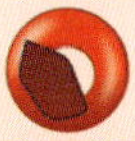	Haemoglobin C disease Haemoglobin SC disease
Red cell agglutinate	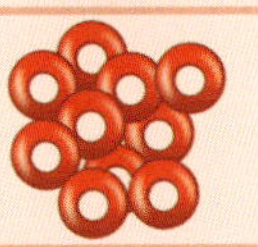	Cold autoimmune haemolytic anaemia Paroxysmal cold haemoglobinuria IgM associated lymphoma Multiple myeloma
Rouleaux	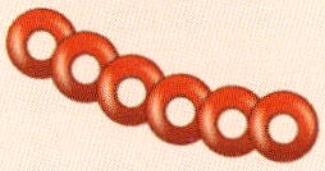	Chronic liver disease malignant lymphoma Multiple myeloma Chronic inflammatory disease

Fig. 2.6: Variation in shape of RBC

Erythropoiesis

DEFINITION

Erythropoiesis is the process of the origin, development and maturation of erythrocytes. Haemopoiesis or haematopoiesis is the process of origin, development and maturation of all the blood cells.

SITE OF ERYTHROPOIESIS (Fig. 3.1)

In Foetal Life

In foetal life, the erythropoiesis occurs in three stages:

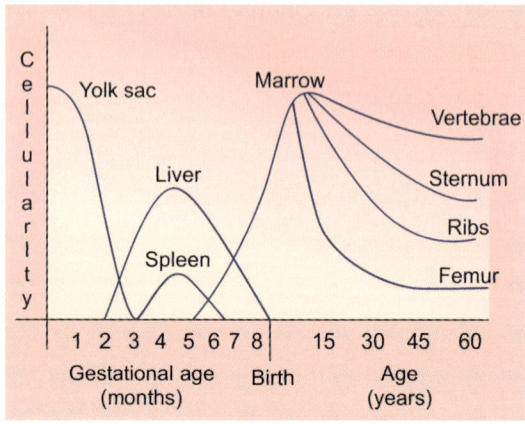

Fig. 3.1: Sites of erythropoiesis according to age

A. Mesoblastic stage

During the first two months of intrauterine life, the RBCs are produced from mesenchyme of yolk sac.

B. Hepatic stage

From third month of intrauterine life, liver is the main organ that produces RBCs. Spleen and lymphoid organs are also involved in erythropoiesis.

C. Myeloid stage

During the last three months of intrauterine life, the RBCs are produced from red bone marrow and liver.

In Newborn Babies, Children and Adults

In newborn babies, growing children and adults, RBCs are produced only from the red bone marrow.

1. **Up to the age of 20 years:** RBCs are produced from red bone marrow of all bones (long bones and all the flat bones).

2. **After the age of 20 years:** RBCs are produced from membranous bones like vertebra, sternum, ribs, scapula, iliac bones and skull bones and from the ends of long bones. After 20 years of age, the shaft of the long bones becomes yellow bone marrow because of fat deposition and looses the erythropoietic function. In adults, liver and spleen may manufacture the blood cells if the bone marrow is destroyed or fibrosed. Collectively bone marrow is almost equal to liver in size and weight. It is also as active as liver. Though bone marrow is the site of production of all blood cells, comparatively 75% of the bone marrow is involved in the production of leukocytes and only 25% is involved in the production of erythrocytes. But still, the leukocytes are less in number than the erythrocytes, the ratio being 1 : 500. This is solely because of the lifespan of these cells. Lifespan of erythrocytes is 120 days whereas the lifespan of leukocytes is very. Short-ranging from one to ten days. So the leukocytes need larger production than erythrocytes to maintain the required number. Stem cells are the primary cells capable of self-renewal and differentiating into specialised cells. Haemopoietic stem cells are the primitive cells in the bone marrow, which give rise to the blood cells. Haemopoietic stem cells in the bone marrow are named uncommitted pluripotent haemopoietic stem cells (PHSC). PHSC is defined as a cell that can give rise to all types of blood cells. In early stages, the PHSC are not designed to form a particular type of blood cell. And it is also not possible to determine the blood cell to be developed from these cells: hence, the name uncommitted PHSC. In adults, only a few number of these cells are present. But the best source of these cells is the umbilical cord blood. When the cells are designed to form a particular type of blood cell, the uncommitted PHSCs are called committed PHSCs. Committed PHSC is defined as a cell, which is restricted to give rise to one group of blood cells.

Committed PHSCs are of two types (Fig. 3.2)

1. Lymphoid stem cells (LSC) which give rise to lymphocytes and natural killer (NK) cells.
2. Colony forming blastocytes, which give rise to myeloid cells. Myeloid cells are the blood cells other than lymphocytes. When grown in cultures, these cells form colonies hence the name colony forming blastocytes.

Different units of colony forming cells are

i. Colony forming unit-erythrocytes (CFU-E)—Cells of this unit develop into erythrocytes.
ii. Colony forming unit-granulocytes/monocytes (CFU-GM)—These cells give rise to granulocytes (neutrophils, basophils and eosinophils) and monocytes.
iii. Colony forming unit-megakaryocytes (CFU-M)—Platelets are developed from these cells.

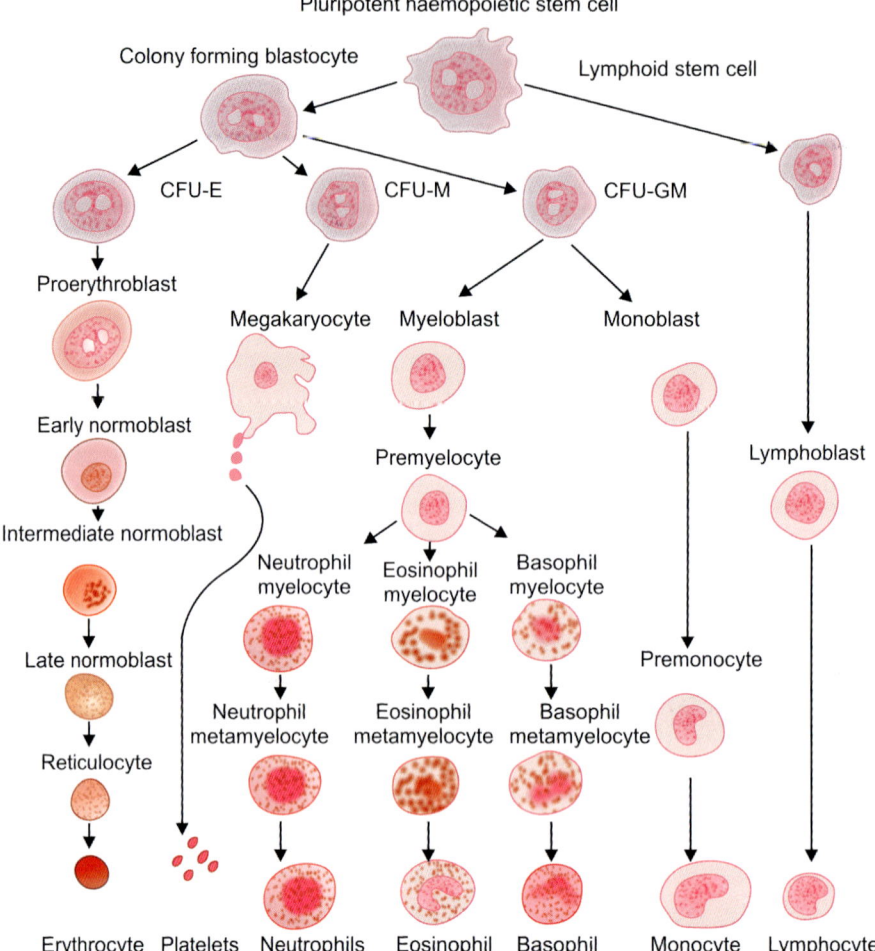

Fig. 3.2: Blood cell lineage

Changes During Erythropoiesis

Cells of CFU-E pass through different stages and finally become the matured RBCs. During these stages four important changes are noticed.

1. Reduction in size of the cell (from the diameter of 25 to 7.2 µm).
2. Disappearance of nucleoli and nucleus.
3. Appearance of haemoglobin.
4. Change in the staining properties of the cytoplasm.

STAGES OF ERYTHROPOIESIS

Various stages (Fig. 3.3) between CFU-E cells and matured RBCs are:

1. Proerythroblast.
2. Early normoblast.
3. Intermediate normoblast.

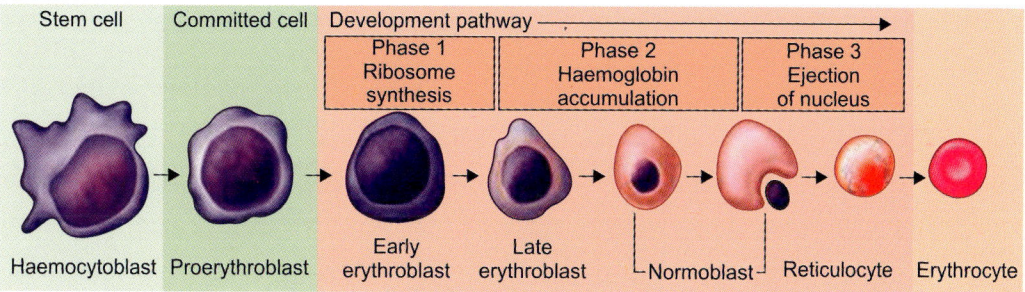

Fig. 3.3: *Stages of erythropoiesis*

4. Late normoblast.
5. Reticulocyte.
6. Matured erythrocyte.

Proerythroblast (Megaloblast)

Proerythroblast (Fig. 3.4) or megaloblast is the first cell derived from CFU-E. It is very large in size with a diameter of about 20 μm. Its nucleus is large and occupies the cell almost completely. The nucleus has two or more nucleoland a reticular network. Proerythroblast does not contain haemoglobin. The cytoplasm is basophilic in nature. Proerythroblast multiplies several times and finally forms the cell of next stage called early normoblast. Synthesis of haemoglobin starts in this stage. However, appearance of haemoglobin occurs only in intermediate normoblast.

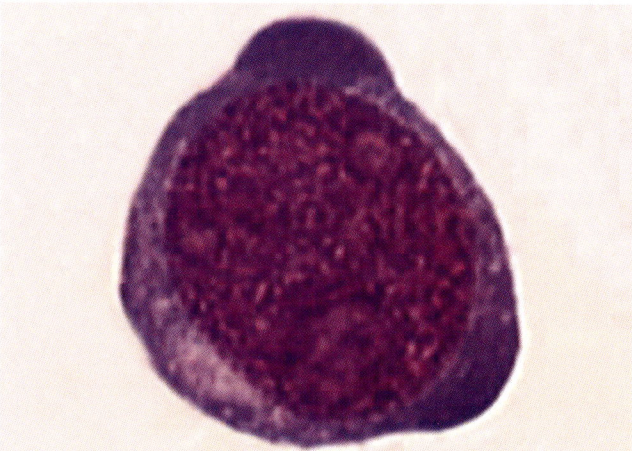

Fig. 3.4: *Proerythroblast*

Early Normoblast

The early normoblast (Fig. 3.5) is small than proerythroblast with a diameter of about 15 μm. In the nucleus, the nucleoli disappear. Condensation of chromatin network occurs. The condensed network becomes dense. The cytoplasm is basophilic in nature. So, this cell is also called basophilic erythroblast. This cell develops into next stage called intermediate normoblast.

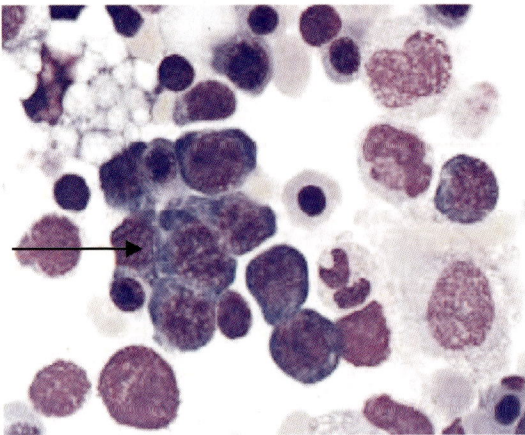

Fig. 3.5: Early normoblast

Intermediate Normoblast (Fig. 3.6)

Cell is smaller than the early normoblast with a diameter of 10 to 12 μm. The nucleus is still present. But, the chromatin network shows further condensation. The haemoglobin starts appearing. Cytoplasm is already basophilic. Now, attributable to the presence of haemoglobin, it stains with both acidic as well as basic stains. So this cell is called polychromophilic or polychromatic erythroblast. This cell develops into next stage called late normoblast.

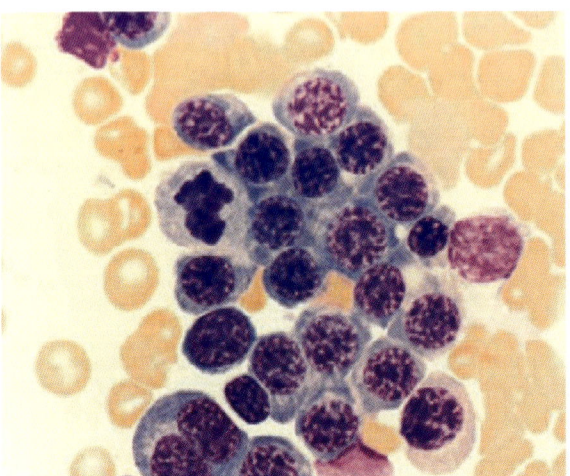

Fig. 3.6: Intermediate normoblast

Late Normoblast (Fig. 3.7)

Diameter of the cell decreases further to about 8 to 10 μm. Nucleus becomes very small with significantly condensed chromatin network and is reffered to as ink-spot nucleus. Quantity of haemoglobin increases. And the cytoplasm becomes almost acidophilic. So, the cell is now called orthochromic erythroblast. In the final stage of late normoblast just before it passes to next stage, the nucleus disintegrates and disappears. The

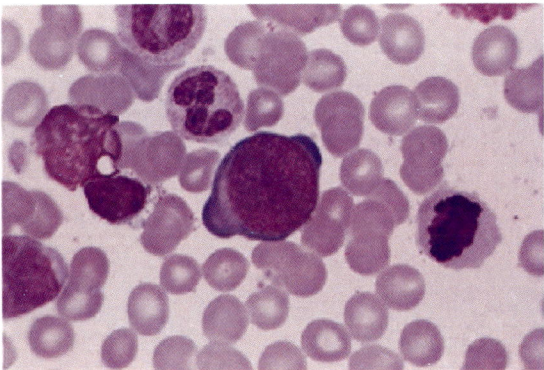

Fig. 3.7: Late normoblast

process by which nucleus disappears is known as pyknosis. The final remnant is extruded from the cell. Late normoblast develops into the next stage known as reticulocyte.

Reticulocyte

Reticulocyte (Fig. 3.8) is otherwise known as immature RBC. It is slightly larger than matured RBC. The cytoplasm contains the reticular network or reticulum, which is formed by remnants of disintegrated organelles. Due to the reticular network, the cell is called reticulocyte. The reticulum of reticulocyte stains with supravital stain.

In newborn babies, the reticulocyte count is 2–6% of RBCs, i.e. 2 to 6 reticulocytes are present for every 100 RBCs. The number of reticulocytes decrease during the first week after birth. Later, the reticulocyte count remains constant at or below 1% of RBCs. The number increases whenever production and release of RBCs increase.

Reticulocyte is basophilic due to the presence of remnants of disintegrated Golgi apparatus, mitochondria and other organelles of cytoplasm. During this stage, the cells enter the blood capillaries through capillary membrane from site of production by diapedesis.

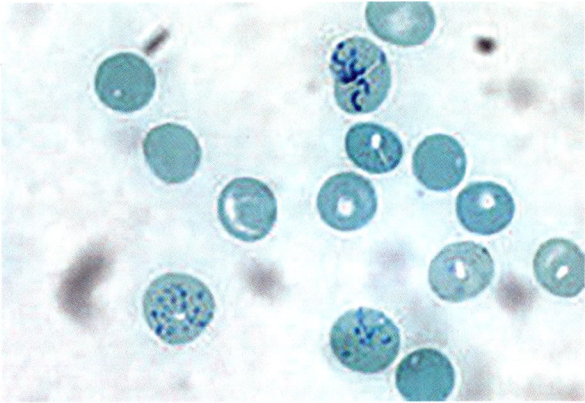

Fig. 3.8: Reticulocyte

Matured Erythrocyte

Reticular network disappears and the cell becomes the matured RBC and attains the biconcave shape. The cell decreases in size to 7.2 µm diameter. The matured RBC is with haemoglobin but without nucleus.

It needs 7 days for the development and maturation of RBC from proerythroblast. It needs 5 days up to the stage of reticulocyte. Reticulocyte takes 2 more days to become the matured RBC.

FACTORS NECESSARY FOR ERYTHROPOIESIS

Development and maturation of erythrocytes require variety of factors, which are classified into three categories:
1. General factors.
2. Maturation factors.
3. Factors necessary for haemoglobin formation.

General Factors

General factors necessary for erythropoiesis are:
 i. Erythropoietin.
 ii. Thyroxine.
 iii. Haemopoietic growth factors.
 iv. Vitamins.

i. Erythropoietin

Most important general factor for erythropoiesis is the hormone called erythropoietin. It is also called haemopoietin or erythrocyte stimulating factor.

Chemistry

Erythropoietin is a glycoprotein with 165 amino acids.

Source of Secretion

Major quantity of erythropoietin is secreted by peritubular capillaries of kidney. A small amount is additionally secreted from liver and brain.

Stimulant for Secretion

Hypoxia is the stimulant for the secretion of erythropoietin.

Actions of Erythropoietin

Erythropoietin causes formation and unleash of latest RBCs into circulation. After secretion, it takes 4 to 5 days to show the action.

Erythropoietin promotes the following processes

 a. Production of proerythroblasts from CFU-E of the bone marrow.
 b. Development of proerythroblasts into matured.
  RBCs through the several stages—early normoblast, intermediate normoblast, late normoblast and reticulocyte
 c. Release of matured erythrocytes into blood. Even some reticulocytes (immature erythrocytes) are released along with matured RBCs. Blood level of erythropoietin increases in anaemia.

ii. Thyroxine

Being a general metabolic hormone, thyroxine accelerates the process of erythropoiesis at many levels. So, hyperthyroidism and polycythemia are common.

iii. Haemopoietic Growth Factors

Haemopoietic growth factors or growth inducers are the interleukins and stem cell factor (steel factor). Generally these factors induce the proliferation of PHSCs. Interleukins (IL) are glycoproteins, which belong to the cytokines family. Interleukins involved in erythropoiesis:

  a. Interleukin-3 (IL-3) secreted by T-cells.
  b. Interleukin-6 (IL-6) secreted by T-cells, endothelial cells and macrophages.
  c. Interleukin-11 (IL-11) secreted by osteoblast.

iv. Vitamins

Some vitamins are also necessary for the process of erythropoiesis. Deficiency of these vitamins cause anaemia associated with other disorders.

Vitamins necessary for erythropoiesis

  a. *Vitamin B*: Its deficiency causes anaemia and pellagra (disease characterised by skin lesions, diarrhoea, weakness, nervousness and dementia).
  b. *Vitamin C*: Its deficiency causes anaemia and scurvy (ancient disease characterised by impaired collagen synthesis resulting in rough skin, bleeding gum, loosening of teeth, poor wound healing, bone pain, lethargy and emotional changes).
  c. *Vitamin D*: Its deficiency causes anaemia and rickets.
  d. *Vitamin E*: Its deficiency leads to anaemia and malnutrition.

MATURATION FACTORS

Vitamin B_{12}, intrinsic factor and folic acid are necessary for the maturation of RBCs.

1. Vitamin B_{12} (Cyanocobalamin)

Vitamin B_{12} is the maturation factor necessary for erythropoiesis.

Source vitamin B_{12} is called extrinsic factor since it is obtained mostly from diet. Its absorption from intestine requires the presence of intrinsic factor of Castle. Vitamin B_{12} is stored mostly in liver and in small quantity in muscle. When necessary, it is transported to the bone marrow to promote maturation of RBCs. It is also produced in the large intestine by the intestinal flora.

Action

Vitamin B_{12} is essential for synthesis of DNA in RBCs. Its deficiency leads to failure in maturation of the cell and reduction in the cell division. Also, the cells are larger with fragile and weak cell membrane resulting in macrocytic anaemia. Deficiency of vitamin B_{12} causes pernicious anaemia. So, vitamin B_{12} is called antipernicious factor.

Intrinsic Factor of Castle

Intrinsic factor of castle is produced in gastric mucosa by the parietal cells of the gastric glands. It is essential for the absorption of vitamin B_{12} from intestine. In the absence of intrinsic factor, vitamin B_{12} is not absorbed from intestine. This leads to pernicious anaemia.

Deficiency of intrinsic factor occurs in

i. Severe gastritis.
ii. Ulcer.
iii. Gastrectomy.

Haematinic Principle

Haematinic principle is the principle thought to be produced by the action of intrinsic factor on extrinsic factor. It is also called or antianaemia principle. It is a maturation factor.

Folic acid

Folic acid is also essential for maturation. It is required for the synthesis of DNA. In the absence of folic acid, the synthesis of DNA decreases causing failure of maturation. This leads to anaemia in which the cells are larger and appear in megaloblastic (proerythroblastic) stage. And, anaemia due to folic acid deficiency is called megaloblastic anaemia.

FACTORS NECESSARY FOR HAEMOGLOBIN FORMATION

Various materials are essential for the formation of haemoglobin in the RBCs. Deficiency of these substances decreases the production of haemoglobin leading to anaemia.

Such Factors are

1. **First class proteins and amino acids:** Proteins of high biological value are essential for the formation of haemoglobin. Amino acids derived from these proteins are required for the synthesis of protein part of haemoglobin, i.e. the globin.
2. **Iron:** Necessary for the formation of haeme part of the haemoglobin.
3. **Copper:** Necessary for the absorption of iron from the gastrointestinal tract.
4. **Cobalt and nickel:** These metals are essential for the utilisation of iron during haemoglobin formation.
5. **Vitamins:** Vitamin C, riboflavin, nicotinic acid and pyridoxine are also essential for the formation of haemoglobin.

Haemoglobin

Haemoglobin (Hb) is the iron containing colouring matter of red blood cell (RBC). It is a chromoprotein forming 95% of dry weight of RBC and 30–34% of wet weight. Function of haemoglobin is to carry the respiratory gases, oxygen and carbon dioxide. It also acts as a buffer. Molecular weight of haemoglobin is 68,000.

NORMAL HAEMOGLOBIN CONTENT

Average haemoglobin (Hb) content in blood is 14 to 16 g/dL. However, the value varies depending upon the age and sex of the individual.

Age

At birth: 25 g/dL
After 3rd month: 20 g/dL
After 1 year: 17 g/dL
From puberty onwards: 14 to 16 g/dL

At the time of birth, haemoglobin content is very high because of increased number of RBCs.

Sex

In adult males: 15 g/dL.
In adult females: 14.5 g/dL.

FUNCTIONS OF HAEMOGLOBIN

Transport of Respiratory Gases

Main function of haemoglobin is the transport of respiratory gases:
1. Oxygen from the lungs to tissues.
2. Carbon dioxide from tissues to lungs.

Transport of Oxygen

When oxygen binds with haemoglobin, a physical process called oxygenation occurs, resulting in the formation of oxyhaemoglobin. The iron remains in ferrous state in this compound. Oxyhaemoglobin is an unstable compound and the combination is reversible, i.e. when more oxygen is available, it combines with haemoglobin and whenever oxygen is required, haemoglobin can release oxygen readily. When oxygen is released from oxyhaemoglobin, it is called reduced haemoglobin or ferrohaemoglobin.

Transport of Carbon Dioxide

When carbon dioxide binds with haemoglobin, carbhaemoglobin is formed. It is also an unstable compound and the combination is reversible, i.e. the carbon dioxide can be released from this compound. The affinity of haemoglobin for carbon dioxide is 20 times more than that for oxygen.

Buffer Action

Haemoglobin acts as a buffer and plays an important role in acid base balance.

Structure of Haemoglobin

Haemoglobin is a conjugated protein. It consists of a protein combined with an iron containing pigment. The protein part is globin and the iron containing pigment is haeme (Fig. 4.1). Haeme also forms a part of the structure of myoglobin (oxygen binding pigment in muscles) and neuroglobin (oxygen binding pigment in brain).

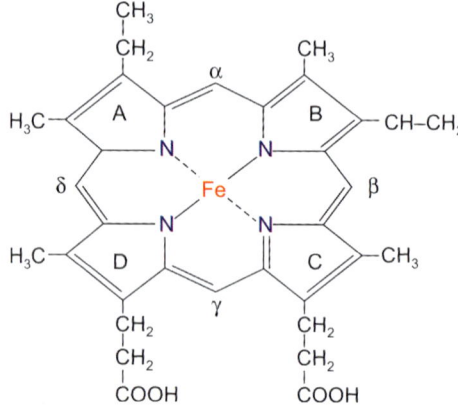

Fig. 4.1: Molecular formula of haeme

Iron

Gold is for the mistress, Silver for the maid
Copper for the Craftsman cunning at his trade
"Good" said the Baron, sitting in the hall,
"But, Iron - Cold Iron, is master of them all".

Rudyard Kipling

Normally, it is present in ferrous (Fe^{2+}) form. It is in unstable or loose form. In some abnormal conditions, the iron is converted into ferric (Fe^{3+}) state, which is a stable form.

Porphyrin

The pigment part of haeme is called porphyrin. It is formed by four pyrrole rings (tetrapyrrole) called, I, II, III and IV. The pyrrole rings are attached to one another by methane (CH_4) bridges. The iron is attached to 'N' of each pyrrole ring and 'N' of globin molecule.

Globin

Globin contains four polypeptide chains. Among the four polypeptide chains, two are alpha and two are beta chains.

Types of Normal Haemoglobin

Haemoglobin is of two types

1. Adult haemoglobin—HbA.
2. Fetal haemoglobin—HbF.

Replacement of fetal haemoglobin by adult haemoglobin starts immediately after birth. It is completed at about 10–12th week after birth. Both the types of haemoglobin differ from each other structurally and functionally.

Structural Difference

In adult haemoglobin, the globin contains two alpha and two beta chains (Fig. 4.2). In fetal haemoglobin, there are two alpha chains and two gamma chains instead of two beta chains.

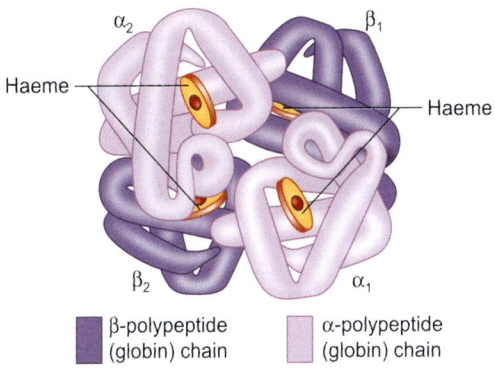

Fig. 4.2: Structure of haemoglobin

Functional Difference

Functionally, fetal haemoglobin has more affinity for oxygen than that of adult haemoglobin. And, the oxygen haemoglobin dissociation curve of fetal blood is shifted to left.

Abnormal Haemoglobin

Abnormal types of haemoglobin or haemoglobin variants are the pathologic mutant forms of haemoglobin. These variants are produced because of structural changes in the polypeptide chains caused by mutation in the genes of the globin chains. Most of the mutations do not produce any serious problem.

Occasionally, few mutations result in some disorders. There are two categories of abnormal haemoglobin:

1. Haemoglobinopathies
2. Haemoglobin in thalassaemia and related disorders.

Haemoglobinopathies

Hemoglobinopathy is a genetic disorder caused by abnormal polypeptide chains of haemoglobin. Some of the haemoglobinopathies are:

 i. *Haemoglobin S*: It is found in sickle cell anaemia. In this, the alpha chains are normal and beta chains are abnormal.

 ii. *Haemoglobin C*: The beta chains are abnormal. It is found in people with haemoglobin C disease, which is characterised by mild haemolytic anaemia and splenomegaly.

 iii. *Haemoglobin E*: Here also the beta chains are abnormal. It is present in people with haemoglobin E disease which is also characterised by mild haemolytic anaemia and splenomegaly.

 iv. *Haemoglobin M*: It is the abnormal haemoglobin present in the form of methaemoglobin. It occurs due to mutation of genes of both in and chains, resulting in abnormal replacement of amino acids.

 It is present in babies affected by haemoglobin M disease or blue baby syndrome. It is an inherited disease, characterised by methaemoglobinemia.

Haemoglobin in Thalassaemia and Related Disorders

In thalassaemia, different types of abnormal haemoglobins are present. The polypeptide chains are decreased, absent or abnormal. In β thalassaemia, the β chains are decreased, absent or abnormal and in β thalassaemia, the β chains are decreased, absent or abnormal. Some of the abnormal haemoglobins found in thalassaemia are haemoglobin G, H, I, Bart's, Kenya, sLepore and constant spring.

Abnormal Haemoglobin Derivatives

'Haemoglobin derivatives' refer to a blood test to detect and measure the percentage of abnormal haemoglobin derivatives. Haemoglobin is the only carrier for transport of oxygen, without which tissue death occurs within few minutes. When haemoglobin is altered, its oxygen carrying capacity is decreased resulting in lack of oxygen. So, it is important to know about the causes and the effects of abnormal haemoglobin derivatives. Abnormal haemoglobin derivatives are formed by carbon monoxide (CO) poisoning or due to some drugs like nitrites, nitrates and sulphonamides.

Abnormal haemoglobin derivatives are

1. Carboxyhaemoglobin.
2. Methaemoglobin.
3. Sulfhaemoglobin.

Normal percentage of haemoglobin derivatives in total haemoglobin:

Carboxyhaemoglobin: 3 to 5 %

Methaemoglobin: Less than 3%

Sulfhaemoglobin: Lrace (undetectable).

   Abnormally high levels of haemoglobin derivates in blood produce serious effects. These derivatives prevent the transport of oxygen resulting in oxygen lack in tissues, which may be fatal.

1. Carboxyhaemoglobin

Carboxyhaemoglobin or carbon monoxyhaemoglobin is the abnormal haemoglobin derivative formed by the combination of carbon monoxide with haemoglobin. Carbon monoxide is a colourless and odourless gas. Since haemoglobin has 200 times more affinity for carbon monoxide than oxygen, it hinders the transport of oxygen resulting in tissue hypoxia. Normally, 1–3% of haemoglobin is in the form of carboxyhaemoglobin.

Sources of Carbon Monoxide

1. Charcoal burning.
2. Coal mines.
3. Deep wells.
4. Underground drainage system.
5. Exhaust of gasoline engines.
6. Gases from guns and other weapons.
7. Heating system with poor or improper ventilation.
8. Smoke from fire.
9. Tobacco smoking.

2. Methaemoglobin

Methaemoglobin is the abnormal haemoglobin derivative formed when iron molecule of haemoglobin is oxidised from normal ferrous state to ferric state. Methaemoglobin is also called ferrihaemoglobin. Normal methaemoglobin level is 0.6–2.5% of total haemoglobin.

Under normal circumstances also, body faces the threat of continuous production of methaemoglobin. But it is counteracted by erythrocyte protective system called nicotinamide adenine dinucleotide (NADH) system, which operates through two enzymes:

1. Diaphorase I (nicotinamide adenine dinucleotide phosphate [NADPH] dependent reductase): Responsible for 95% of the action.
2. Diaphorase II (NADPH dependent methaemoglobin reductase): Responsible for 5% of the action. These two enzymes prevent the oxidation of ferrous iron into ferric iron.

Methaemoglobinemia

Methaemoglobinemia is the disorder characterised by high level of methaemoglobin in blood.

It leads to tissue hypoxia, which causes cyanosis and other symptoms.

Causes of Methaemoglobinemia

Methaemoglobinemia is caused by variety of factors:

1. Common factors of daily life

i. Well water contaminated with nitrates and nitrites.
ii. Fires.
iii. Laundry ink.
iv. Match sticks and explosives.
v. Meat preservatives (which contain nitrates and nitrites).
vi. Mothballs (naphthalene balls).
vii. Room deodoriser propellants.

2. Exposure to industrial chemicals such as

    i. Aromatic amines.
    ii. Fluorides.
    iii. Irritant gases like nitrous oxide and nitrobenzene.
    iv. Propylene glycol dinitrate.

3. Drugs

    i. Antibacterial drugs like sulfonamides.
    ii. Antimalarial drugs like chloroquine.
    iii. Antiseptics.
    iv. Inhalant in cyanide antidote kit.
    v. Local anaesthetics like benzocaine.

4. Hereditary trait

Due to deficiency of NADH-dependant reductase or presence of abnormal haemoglobin M. Haemoglobin M is common in babies affected by blue baby syndrome (a pathological condition in infants, characterised by bluish skin discolouration (cyanosis), caused by congenital heart defect).

3. Sulfhaemoglobin

Sulfhaemoglobin is the abnormal haemoglobin derivative, formed by the combination of haemoglobin with hydrogen sulphide. It is caused by drugs such as phenacetin or sulfonamides. Normal sulfhaemoglobin level is less than 1% of total haemoglobin. Sulfhaemoglobin cannot be converted back into haemoglobin. Only way to get rid of this from the body is to wait until the affected RBCs with sulfhaemoglobin are destroyed after their lifespan.

Blood Level of Sulfhaemoglobin

Normally, very negligible amount of sulfhaemoglobin is present in blood which is nondetectable. But when its level rises above 10 gm/dL, cyanosis occur. Usually, serious toxic effects are not noticed.

Synthesis of Haemoglobin

Synthesis of haemoglobin actually starts in proerythroblastic stage. However, haemoglobin appears in the intermediate normoblastic stage only. Production of haemoglobin is continued until the stage of reticulocyte. Haeme portion of haemoglobin is synthesised in mitochondria. And the protein part, globin is synthesised in ribosomes.

Synthesis of Haeme

Haeme is synthesised from succinylCoA and the glycine. The sequence of events in synthesis of haemoglobin (Fig. 4.3):

1. First step in haeme synthesis takes place in the mitochondrion. Two molecules of succinylCoA combine with two molecules of glycine and condense to form-aminolevulinic acid (ALA) by ALA synthase.

2. ALA is transported to the cytoplasm. Two molecules of ALA combine to form porphobilinogen in the presence of ALA dehydratase.

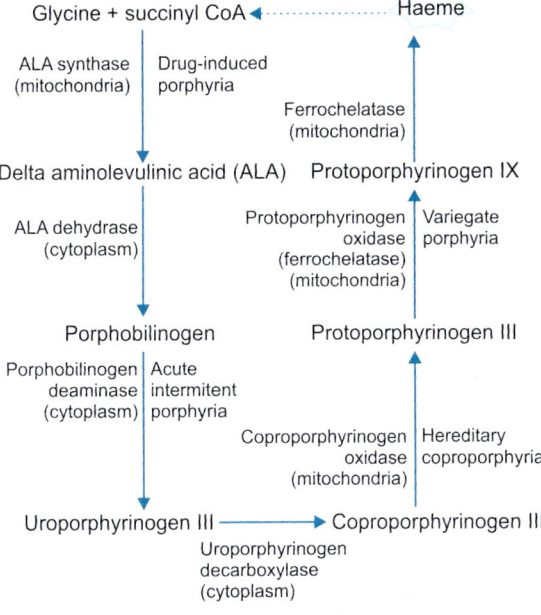

Fig. 4.3: Haeme synthesis

3. Porphobilinogen is converted into uroporphobilinogen I by uroporphobilinogen I synthase.
4. Uroporphobilinogen I is converted into uropor phobilinogen III by porphobilinogen III cosynthase.
5. From uroporphobilinogen III, a ring structure called coproporphyrinogen III is formed by uroporphobilinogen decarboxylase.
6. Coproporphyrinogen III is transported back to the mitochondrion, where it is oxidised to form protoporphyrinogen IX by coproporphyrinogen oxidase.
7. Protoporphyrinogen IX is converted into protoporphyrin IX by protoporphyrinogen oxidase.
8. Protoporphyrin IX combines with iron to form haeme in the presence of ferrochelatase.

Formation of Globin

Polypeptide chains of globin are produced in the ribosomes. There are four types of polypeptide chains namely, alpha, beta, gamma and delta chains. Each of these chains differs from others by the amino acid sequence. Each globin molecule is formed by the combination of 2 pairs of chains and each chain is made of 141 to 146 amino acids. Adult haemoglobin contains two alpha chains and two beta chains. Fetal haemoglobin contains two alpha chains and two gamma chains.

Configuration

Each polypeptide chain combines with one haeme molecule. Thus, after the complete configuration, each haemoglobin molecule contains four polypeptide chains and four haeme molecules.

Haemoglobin Metabolism

After the lifespan of 120 days, the RBC is destroyed in the reticuloendothelial system, particularly in spleen and the haemoglobin is released into plasma. Soon, the haemoglobin is degraded in the reticuloendothelial cells and split into globin and haeme. Globin is utilised for the resynthesis of haemoglobin. Heme is degraded into iron and porphyrin (Fig. 4.4). Iron is stored in the body as ferritin and haemosiderin, which are reutilised for the synthesis of new haemoglobin. Porphyrin is converted into a green pigment called biliverdin. In human being, most of the biliverdin is converted into a yellow pigment called bilirubin. Bilirubin and biliverdin are together called the bile pigments.

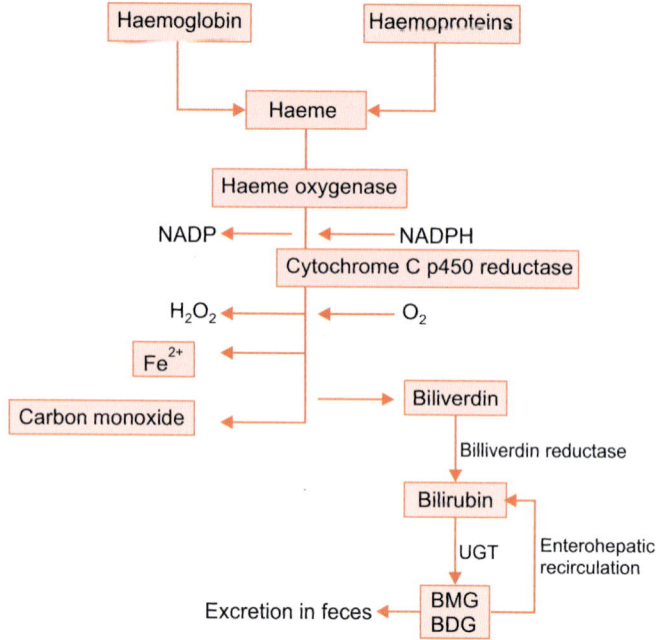

Fig. 4.4: Heme metabolism

Iron Metabolism (Fig. 4.5)

Iron is an essential mineral and an important component of proteins, involved in oxygen transport. So, human body needs iron for oxygen transport. Iron is important for the formation of haemoglobin and myoglobin. Iron is also necessary for the formation of other substances like cytochrome, cytochrome oxidase, peroxidase and catalase.

NORMAL VALUE AND DISTRIBUTION OF IRON IN THE BODY

Total quantity of iron in the body is about 4 gm. Approximate distribution of iron in the body is as follows:

In the haemoglobin: 65–68%

In the muscle as myoglobin: 4%

As intracellular oxidative haeme compound: 1%

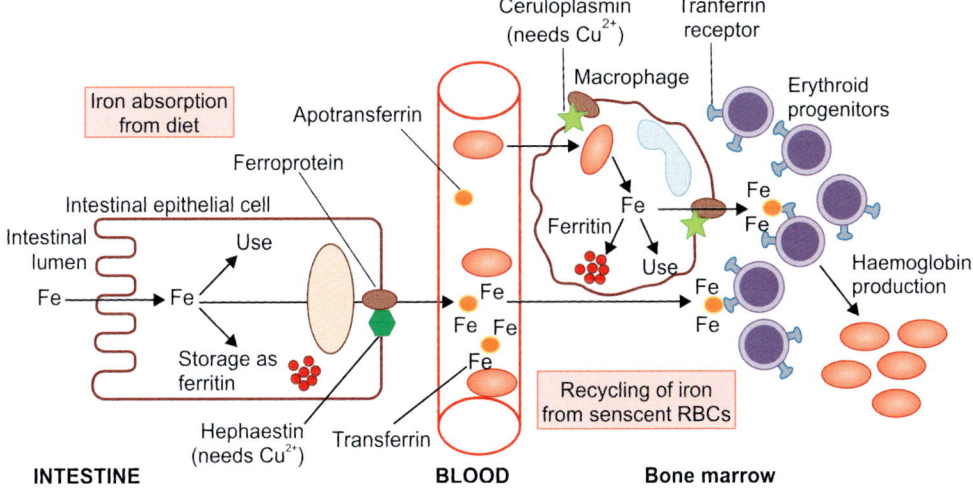

Fig. 4.5: Iron metabolism

In the plasma as transferrin: 0.1%
Stored in the reticuloendothelial system: 25–30%.

DIETARY IRON

Dietary iron (Fig. 4.6) is available in two forms called haeme and nonhaeme.

Haeme Iron

Haeme iron is present in fish, meat and chicken. Iron in these sources is found in the form of haeme. Haeme iron is absorbed easily from intestine.

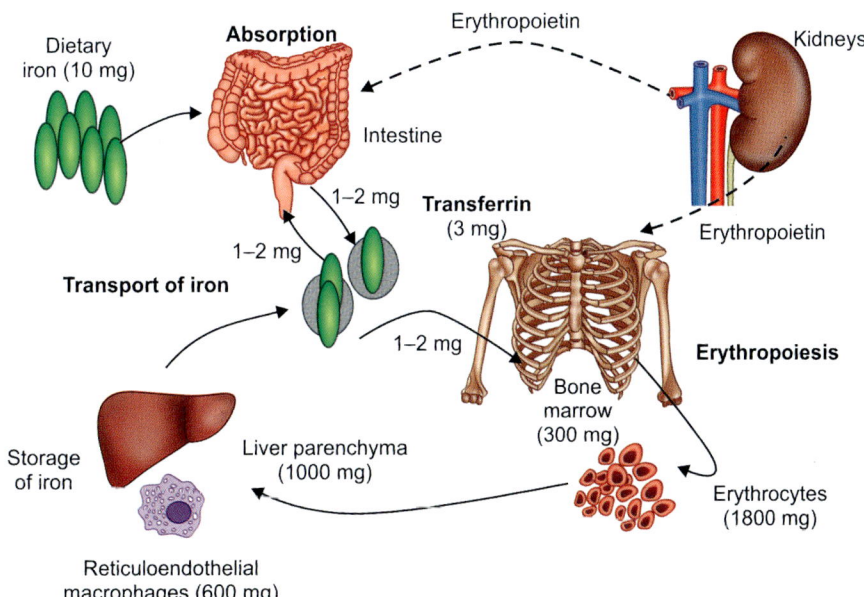

Fig. 4.6: Fate of dietary iron

Nonhaeme Iron

Iron in the form of nonhaeme is available in vegetables, grains and cereals. Nonhaeme iron is not absorbed easily as haeme iron. Cereals, flours and products of grains which are enriched or fortified (strengthened) with iron become good dietary sources of nonhaeme iron, particularly for children and women.

ABSORPTION OF IRON

Iron is absorbed mainly from the small intestine (Fig. 4.7). It is absorbed through the intestinal cells (enterocytes) by pinocytosis and transported into the blood. Bile is essential for the absorption of iron.

Iron is present mostly in ferric (Fe^{3+}) form. It is converted into ferrous form (Fe^{2+}) which is absorbed into the blood. Hydrochloric acid from gastric juice makes the ferrous iron soluble so that it could be converted into ferric iron by the enzyme ferric reductase from enterocytes. From enterocytes, ferric iron is transported into blood by a protein called ferroprotein. In the blood, ferric iron is converted into ferrous iron and transported.

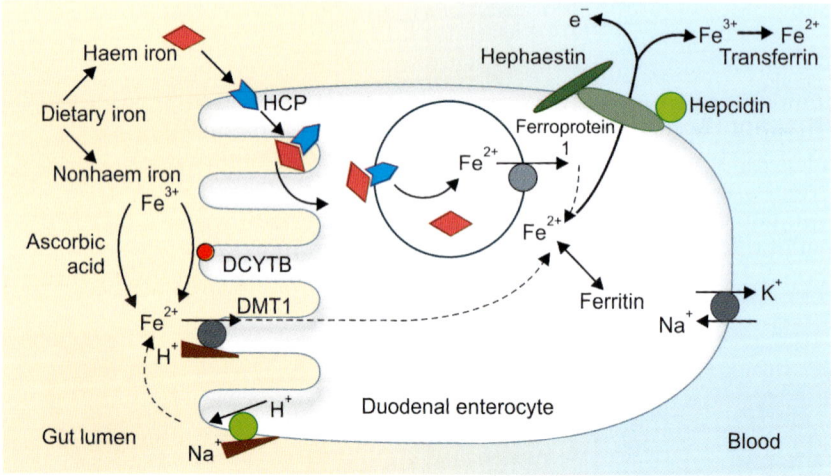

Fig. 4.7: Iron absorption

TRANSPORT OF IRON

Immediately after absorption into blood, iron combines with β-globulin called apotransferrin (secreted by liver through bile) resulting in the formation of transferrin. And iron is transported in blood in the form of transferring (Fig. 4.8). Iron combines loosely with globin and can be released easily at any region of the body.

STORAGE OF IRON

Iron is stored in large quantities in reticuloendothelial cells and liver hepatocytes. In other cells also it is stored in small quantities. In the cytoplasm of the cell, iron is stored as ferritin in large amount. Small quantity of iron is also stored as haemosiderin.

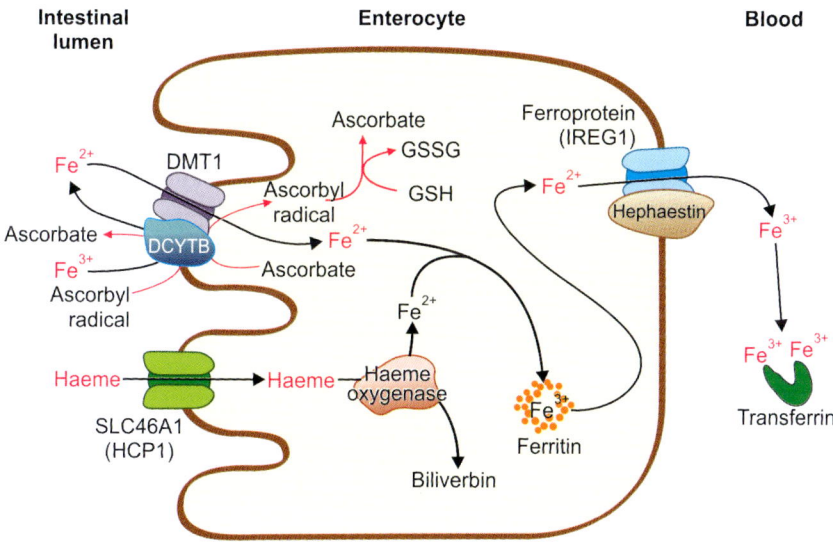

Fig. 4.8: Transport of iron

DAILY LOSS OF IRON

In males, about 1 mg of iron is excreted everyday through faeces. In females, the amount of iron loss is very much high. This is because of the menstruation. One gram of haemoglobin contains 3.34 mg of iron.

Normally, 100 mL of blood contains 15 gm of haemoglobin and about 50 mg of iron (3.34 × 15). So, if 100 mL of blood is lost from the body, there is a loss of about 50 mg of iron. In females, during every menstrual cycle, about 50 mL of blood is lost by which 25 mg of iron is lost. This is why the iron content is always less in females than in males.

Iron is lost during haemorrhage and blood donation also. If 450 mL of blood is donated, about 225 mg of iron is lost.

REGULATION OF TOTAL IRON IN THE BODY

Absorption and excretion of iron are maintained almost equally under normal physiological conditions. When the iron storage is saturated in the body, it automatically reduces the further absorption of iron from the gastrointestinal tract by feedback mechanism.

Factors which reduce the absorption of iron

1. Stoppage of apotransferrin formation in the liver, so that the iron cannot be absorbed from the intestine.
2. Reduction in the release of iron from the transferrin, so that transferrin is completely saturated with iron and further absorption is prevent.

Haematological Changes in Pregnancy

RBC

During pregnancy, the total blood volume increases by about 1.5 liters, mainly to supply the demands of the new vascular bed and to compensate for blood loss occurring at delivery. Of this, around one liter of blood is contained within the uterus and maternal blood spaces of the placenta. Increase in blood volume is, therefore, more marked in multiple pregnancies and in iron deficient states. Expansion of plasma volume occurs by 10–15 % at 6–12 weeks of gestation. During pregnancy, plasma renin activity tends to increase and atrial natriuretic peptide levels tend to reduce, though slightly. This suggests that, in pregnant state, the elevation in plasma volume is in response to an underfilled vascular system resulting from systemic vasodilatation and increase in vascular capacitance, rather than actual blood volume expansion, which would produce the opposite hormonal profile instead (i.e. low plasma renin and elevated atrial natriuretic peptide levels).

Red cell mass (driven by an increase in maternal erythropoietin production) also increases, but relatively less, compared with the increase in plasma volume, the net result being a dip in haemoglobin concentration. Thus, there is dilutional anaemia. The drop in haemoglobin is typically by 1–2 gm/dL by the late second trimester and stabilises thereafter in the third trimester, when there is a reduction in maternal plasma volume (owing to an increase in levels of atrial natriuretic peptide). Women who take iron supplements have less pronounced changes in haemoglobin, as they increase their red cell mass in a more proportionate manner than those not on haematinic supplements.

The red blood cell indices change little in pregnancy. However, there is a small increase in mean corpuscular volume (MCV), of an average of 4 fl in an iron-replete woman, which reaches a maximum at 30–35 weeks gestation and does not suggest any deficiency of vitamins B_{12} and folate. Increased production of RBCs to meet the demands of pregnancy, reasonably explains why there is an increased MCV (due to a higher proportion of young RBCs which are larger in size). However, MCV does not change significantly during pregnancy and a haemoglobin concentration <9.5 gm/dL in association with a mean corpuscular volume <84 fl probably indicates coexistent iron deficiency or some other pathology.

Postpregnancy, plasma volume decreases as a result of diuresis, and the blood volume returns to nonpregnant values. Haemoglobin and haematocrit increase consequently. Plasma volume increases again two to five days later, possibly because of a rise in aldosterone secretion. Later, it again decreases. Significant elevation has been documented between measurements of haemoglobin taken at 6–8 weeks postpartum and those taken at 4–6 months postpartum, indicating that it takes at least

4–6 months postpregnancy, to restore the physiological dip in haemoglobin to the non-pregnant values.

WBC

White blood cell count is increased in pregnancy with the lower limit of the reference range being typically 6,000/cmm. Leucocytosis, occurring during pregnancy is due to the physiologic stress induced by the pregnant state. Neutrophils are the major type of leucocytes on differential counts. This is likely due to impaired neutrophilic apoptosis in pregnancy. The neutrophil cytoplasm shows toxic granulation. Neutrophil chemotaxis and phagocytic activity are depressed, especially due to inhibitory factors present in the serum of a pregnant female. There is also evidence of increased oxidative metabolism in neutrophils during pregnancy. Immature forms as myelocytes and metamyelocytes may be found in the peripheral blood film of healthy women during pregnancy and do not have any pathological significance. They simply indicate adequate bone marrow response to an increased drive for erythropoiesis occurring during pregnancy.

Lymphocyte count decreases during pregnancy through the first and second trimesters and increases during the third trimester. There is an absolute monocytosis during pregnancy, especially in the first trimester, but decreases as gestation advances. Monocytes help in preventing foetal allograft rejection by infiltrating the decidual tissue (7–20th week of gestation) possibly, through PGE_2 mediated immunosuppression. The monocyte to lymphocyte ratio is markedly increased in pregnancy. Eosinophil and basophil counts, however, do not change significantly during pregnancy.

The stress of delivery may itself lead to brisk leucocytosis. Few hours after delivery, healthy women have been documented as having a WBC count varying from 9,000 to 25,000/cmm. By four weeks postdelivery, typical WBC ranges are similar to those in healthy nonpregnant women.

Pregnancy is a hypercoaguable condition where characteristic changes appear in coagulation profile too (Table. 5.1).

Table 5.1: Changes in clotting factor in pregnancy		
Coag factor	*Nonpregnancy*	*Pregnancy*
Fibrinogen	300 mg/dL	450 mg/dL (50%)
Factor VII, VIII, IX, X		Appreciably increased
Factor II		Slightly increased
Factor XI, XII		Slightly decreased
Platelets		Moderate decrease in number (15%)
Clotting time		Not altered

Anaemia in Pregnancy

INTRODUCTION

Anaemia is one of the most commonly encountered medical disorders during pregnancy. In developing countries it is one of the serious concerns, besides many other adverse effects on the mother and the foetus it contributes significantly high maternal mortality. According to United Nation declaration 1997, anaemia is a major public health problem that needs total elimination. It is estimated that globally two billion people suffer from iron deficiency anaemia.

PREVALENCE OF ANAEMIA IN PREGNANCY

According to World Health Organization estimates, up to 56% of all women living in developing countries are anaemic. In India, National Family Health Survey –2 (Fig. 6.1) in 1998 to 99 shows that 54% of women in rural and 46% women in urban areas are anaemics. The prevalence of mild, moderate, and severe anaemia are 13%, 57% and 12% respectively in India (ICMR data). According to WHO, haemoglobin level below 11gm/dL in pregnant women constitutes anaemia and haemoglobin below 7 gm/dL is severe anaemia. The Center for Disease Control and Prevention (1990) defines anaemia as less than 11 gm/dL in the first and third trimester and less than 10.5 gm/dL in second trimester. Serum Ferritin of 15 µg/L is associated with iron deficiency anaemia.

ERYTHROPOIESIS IN PREGNANCY

Different factors required for erythropoiesis are proteins (erythropoietin), minerals (iron), trace elements (including zinc, cobalt and copper), vitamins (particularly folic

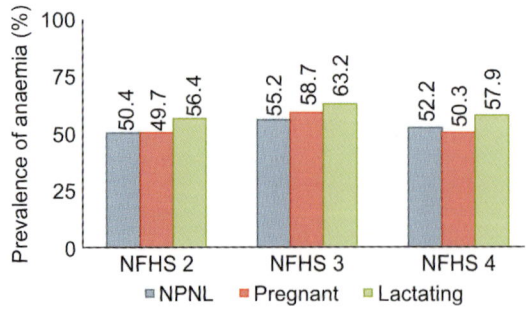

Fig. 6.1: NHFS data

acid, vitamin B_{12} [cyanocobalamin], vitamin C, pyridoxine; and riboflavin), and hormones (androgens and thyroxine).

In addition to the common deficiencies of iron and folate, there is a growing body of evidence to implicate vitamin A (important for cell growth and differentiation maintenance of epithelial integrity and normal immune function) and Zn (important in protein synthesis and nucleic acid metabolism) in nutritional anaemias.

In anaemia there is low circulating haemoglobin (Hb) in which concentration has fallen below a threshold lying at two standard deviations below the median of a healthy population of the same age, sex and stage of pregnancy. The WHO definition for diagnosis of anaemia in pregnancy is a Hb concentration of less than 11 gm/dL (7.45 mmol/L) and a haematocrit of less than 33%.

TYPES OF ANAEMIA

Physiological Anaemia

In pregnancy there is a disproportionate increase in plasma volume, RBC volume and haemoglobin mass. The plasma volume increase more than the RBC mass haemodilution occurs and is called physiological anaemia of pregnancy.

Criteria are

  a. RBC 3.2 million/cmm.
  b. Haemoglobin 10 gm%.
  c. RBC morphology on peripheral smear is normal, i.e. normocytic, normochromic.
  d. PCV 30%.

Pathological Anaemia

WHO definition of Anaemia in Pregnancy

• Haemoglobin less than 11 gm/dL is considered as anaemia.
• In India, FOGSI recommends haemoglobin less than 10 gm/dL during pregnancy is considered as anaemia.

Table 6.1: Classification of anaemia		
	ICMR	*WHO*
Mild	10–11 gm/dL	9–11 gm/dL
Moderate	7–10 gm/dL	7–9 gm/dL
Severe	4–7 gm/dL	<7 gm/dL
Very severe	<4 gm/dL	

CDC definition of Anaemia in Pregnancy

Hb <11 gm/dL uring first and third trimester and <10.5 gm/dL in the second trimester (to allow for the physiological fall due to haemodilution in second trimester).

Iron Deficiency Anaemia

About 1000 mg of iron is required during pregnancy. 500–600 mg for RBC expansion. 300 mg for foetus and placenta and the rest for the growing uterus. As a result of amenorrhoea there is a saving of about 150 mg of iron and therefore, about 850 mg of extra iron is required during pregnancy. Diet alone cannot provide the extra iron and stores which have around 500 mg of iron get depleted. But if iron stores are already deficient, iron deficiency anaemia manifests. Iron deficiency anaemia (IDA) is the commonest type of anaemia in pregnancy.

Iron nutritional status depends on long-term iron balance and is favoured by ingestion of adequate amounts of iron in the diet (native or fortified) or through iron supplementation. The balance is adversely affected by the loss of iron through intestinal mucosal turnover and excretion, skin desquamation, menstruation and lactation. Iron absorption is 15–30% (haem iron) and up to 50% in the iron deficiency state reduce to 5–8% with an excessive haem diet. Its absorption is usually not affected by inhibitors.

The nonhaem iron pool is made of all other sources of iron such as cereals, seeds, vegetables, milk and eggs. Its absorption can be increased by enhancers (haem, proteins, ascorbic acid and fermentation) and decreased by inhibitors (phytic acid, fibres, calcium, tannins, tea, coffee, chocolate and herbal infusion). On the basis of type of food, iron bioavailability can be characterised as follows.

DIET IN RELATION TO NUTRITIONAL ANAEMIA (Fig. 7.1)

Low Bioavailability Diets

Simple diet of beans, whole wheat flour and sorghum with negligible amounts of meat, fish and ascorbic acid. In nonindustrialised countries, a very low bioavailable iron,

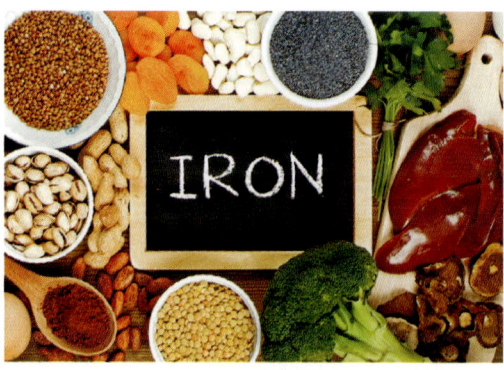

Fig. 7.1: Sources of iron

vegetarian diet low in ascorbic acid and high in biological proteins composed almost entirely of cereals is consumed with excess of inhibitors of iron absorption (phytates); thus, absorption may be as low as 3.4%.

Intermediate Bioavailability Diet

Diets in this category are mainly comprised of cereals, roots or tubers, but include some animal foods like meat, fish and ascorbic acid which increase the iron absorption.

High Bioavailability Diet

This is a varied diet rich in meat, poultry, fish and foods with a generous amount of ascorbic acid, as found in industrialised countries.

WORM INFESTATION

Prevalence of amoebiasis and giardiasis is around 40%. Increased iron loss due to hookworm infestations, schistosomiasis, chronic malaria, excessive sweating and blood loss from the gut due to haemorrhoids are important causes of anaemia in pregnancy.

MULTIPLE PREGNANCIES

Most women enter pregnancy with little or no iron reserve, which is further compounded by repeated and closely spaced pregnancies and prolonged periods of lactation.

EFFECTS OF ANAEMIA ON PREGNANCY

Anaemia has deleterious effects (Fig. 7.2) on mother and the fetus and it turns into a vicious cycle with a adverse outcome.

Maternal Effects

Mild, anaemia may not have any effect on pregnancy and labour except that the mother will have low iron stores and may become moderately to- severely anemic in

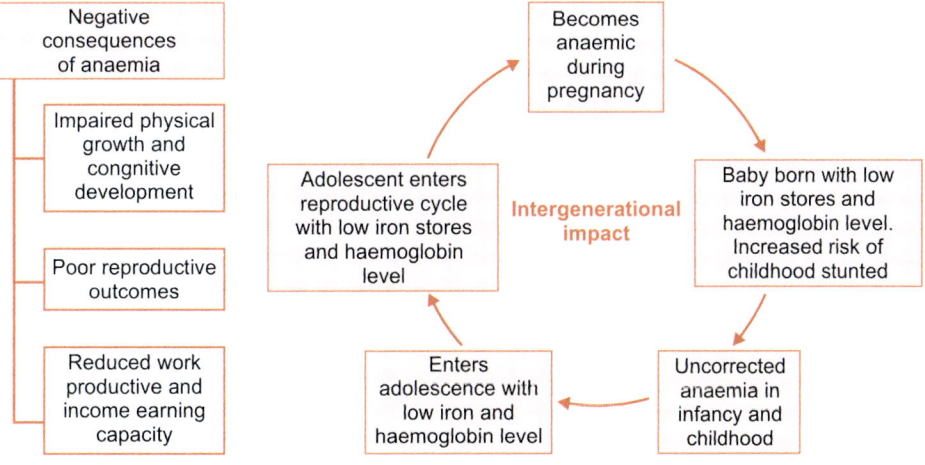

Fig. 7.2: Implication of anaemia

subsequent pregnancies. Moderate anaemia may cause increased weakness, lack of energy, fatigue and poor work performance. Severe anaemia, however, is associated with poor outcome. The woman may have palpitations, tachycardia, breathlessness, increased cardiac output leading onto cardiac stress which can cause decompensation and cardiac failure which may be fatal 5, 8. Increased incidence of preterm labour (28.2%), pre-eclampsia (31.2%) and sepsis have been associated with anaemia.

Foetal Effects

Irrespective of maternal iron stores, the foetus still obtains iron from maternal transferrin, which is trapped in the placenta and which, in turn, removes, and actively transports iron to the foetus. Gradually, however, such foetuses tend to have decreased iron stores due to depletion of maternal stores. Adverse perinatal outcome in the form of preterm and small-forgestational-age babies and increased perinatal mortality rates have been observed in the neonates of anaemic mothers. Iron supplementation to the mother during pregnancy improves perinatal outcome. Mean weight, Apgar score and haemoglobin level 3 month after birth were significantly greater in babies of the supplemented group than the placebo group.

CLINICAL FEATURES OF IRON DEFICIENCY ANAEMIA

Symptoms (Fig. 7.3)

There may be no symptoms, especially in mild and moderate anaemia. Patient may complain of feelings of weakness, exhaustion and lassitude, indigestion and loss of appetite. Palpitation, dyspnoea, giddiness, oedema and, rarely, generalised anasarca and even congestive cardiac failure can occur in severe cases.

Signs

There may be no signs especially in mild anaemia. There may be pallor, glossitis and stomatitis. Patients may have oedema due to hypoproteinaemia. Soft systolic murmur can be heard in mitral area due to hyperdynamic circulation.

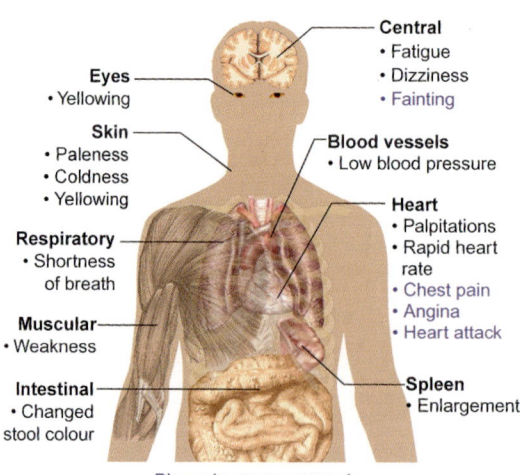

Fig. 7.3: Symptoms of anaemia

Most Critical Period

- 28–30 weeks of pregnancy
- In labour
- Immediately after delivery
- Early puerperium
- CHF (failure to cope up with pregnancy induced cardiac load).

INVESTIGATION

- Severity of anaemia—Hb and haematocrit, at first visit, 28–30 weeks and 36 weeks. Haemoglobin estimation is the most practical method of diagnosis as it is cost effective and can be easily performed by trained technician. Sahil's methods is reliable and accurate when done by expert, and is the most communally used method, although the cyanomethaemoglobin, method appears to be the most accurate.
- Type of anaemia—PBS, microcytic, macrocytic, dimorphic, normocytic, haemolytic, pancytopenia.
- Bone marrow activity—reticulocyte count (N .2–2%), higher bone marrow activity is seen in:
  - Haemolytic anaemia
  - Following acute blood loss
  - Iron deficiency anaemia on treatment.
- Cause of anaemia—by various investigations.

PERIPHERAL BLOOD SMEAR

Normal smear—Normocytic (normal size RBC), normochromic (normal colour RBC) iron deficiency (Fig. 7.4)—Microcytic (small RBC), hypochromic (pale RBC), anisocytosis (variation in size), poikilocytosis (variation in shape), with or without target cells.

Malarial parasites can be seen.

Aplastic anaemia shows low/no count.

Sickle cells can be demonstrated.

Toxic granules can be seen.

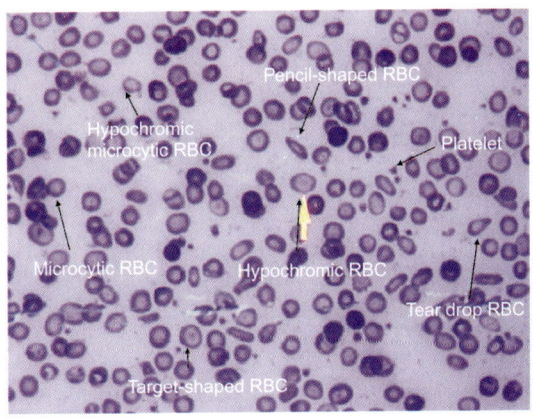

Fig. 7.4: Peripheral blood smear of iron deficiency anaemia

Abnormal blast cells seen in leukemia.

Target cells in thalassaemia.

RBC INDICES

RBC count—decreases in anaemia (N 3.2 million/cmm)

PCV—<32%, (N37–47%)

MCV—Low in Fe deficiency anaemia, microcytic

MCH—Decreases

MCHC—Decreases, one of the most sensitive indices (N26–30%).

Blood indices help in differentiating microcytic anaemia on peripheral blood smear. (Table 7.1).

SPECIAL INVESTIGATION

Serum ferritin—abnormal if < 20 ng/mL (N 40–160 ng/dL), assess iron stores.

Serum tron—N 65–165 µg/dL, decreases in Fe deficiency anaemia.

Serum iron binding capacity—300–360 µg/dL, increases with severity of anaemia.

Percentage saturation of transferrin—35–50%, decreases to less than 20% in fe anaemia. Serum transferrin receptor appears to be specific and sensitive marker of iron deficiency in pregnancy. Its levels are increased in iron deficiency anaemia.

RBC protoporphyrin—30 µg/dL, it doubles or triples in Fe deficiency anaemia (substrate to bind with Fe, cannot be converted into Hb in Fe deficiency).

OTHER INVESTIGATION

Urine examination—RBC and casts

In areas where schistosomiasis is prevalent, urine examination for occult blood and schistosomes should be performed

Stool examination—occult blood, ova

As worm infestations are common causes of anaemia, stool examination for ova and cysts should be done consecutively for three days in all cases

Bone marrow examination—refractory anaemia.

Table 7.1: Difference in laboratory parameters between iron deficiency anaemia and thalassaemia

Parameter	Iron deficiency	α-thalasaemia minor	β-thalasaemia minor
MCV	↓	↓	↓
RDW	↑	Normal	Normal
RBCs	↓	Normal	Normal
Peripheral smear	Nicrocytosis, hypochromia	Target cells	Target cells
Serum iron studies	↓ iron and ferritin ↑ TIBC	Normal/↑ iron and ferritin (RBC turnover)	Normal/↑ iron and ferritin (RBC turnover)
Response to iron supplementation	↑ Haemoglobin	No improvement	No improvement
Haemoglobin electrophoresis	Normal	Normal	↑ Haemoglobin A2

Bone marrow examination by staining with potassium ferrocyanate to see characteristic blue granules of stainable iron in, erythroblasts is the most accurate method for iron stores, but is not practical in most cases as the test is invasive, Bone marrow, examination is only dated in cases where there is no response to iron therapy after 4 weeks or for diagnosis of kala-azar or in suspected aplastic anaemia.

X-Ray chest—Pulmonary TB.

BUN/Serum creatinine—Renal disease.

After anaemia typing on peripheral blood smear still there is need to perform few more laboratory investigations for definitive diagnosis of anaemia (Fig. 7.5).

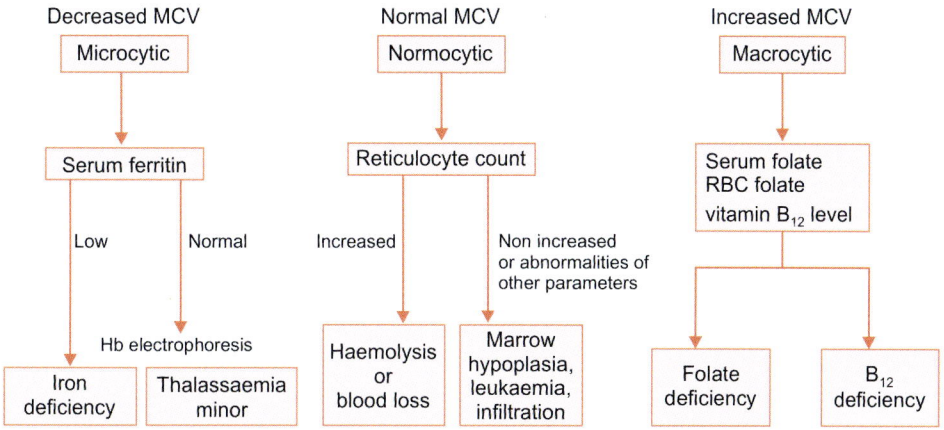

Fig. 7.5: Stepwise differentiation strategy for anaemia after peripheral smear

MANAGEMENT

Prevention of Iron Deficiency

Prophylaxis of Nonpregnant Women

As most women start their pregnancy with anaemia or low iron stores, so prevention should start even before pregnancy. As a public health approach, prolonged oral supplementation beginning before the woman becomes pregnant may be a better strategy to benefit the majority of the population. Twelve by twelve initiative is one such initiative aiming to have Hb of 12 gm/dL by 12 year of age using prophylactic iron therapy and advising consumption of iron rich food.

Iron supplementation by 30 doses administered weekly over 7 months was as effective as 90 doses consumed daily for 3 months. Hence, women of childbearing age in developing countries should receive a 2–4 months course of 60 mg of iron daily. In addition, concomitant use of folate will prevent neural tube defects in the newborn.

Iron Supplementation During Pregnancy

The Ministry of Health, Government of India has now recommended intake of 100 mg of elemental iron with 500 mg of folic acid in the second half of pregnancy for a period of at least 100 days. Women who receive daily antenatal iron supplementation are less likely to have iron deficiency anaemia at term. Even two injection of iron dextran

(250 mg each) given intramuscularly at 4 week intervals along with tetanus toxoid injection have been recommended for better compliance and adequate results.

Treatment of Hookworm Infestation

As worm infestation is very common and given the safety of the deworming drugs, oral antihelminthic treatment can also be given to pregnant and lactating women. Single albendazole (400 mg) or mebendazole (100 mg) doses twice daily for 3 days with iron supplementation should be given to all anaemic pregnant; women in the second and third trimesters for better results.

Improvement of Dietary Habits and Improving the Bioavailability of Food Iron

Those pregnant should eat foods rich in iron (jaggery, green leafy vegetables like spinach, mustard leaves, turnip green, cereals, and sprouted pulses) cook their food in iron utensils. Too much of cooking should be avoided.

Social Services

Improvement of sanitation, personal hygiene, better education and alleviation of poverty are not easy tasks and need political will also.

Food Fortification

Iron fortification of foods is a preventive measure that aims at improving and sustaining iron nutrition on a permanent basis. Even common salt, which is often fortified successfully with iodine in deficient areas, can be fortified with iron as has been successfully done in various South-East Asian and Latin American countries. Production of iron fortified salt on a commercial scale has been approved by the Government of India and is in the process of manufacture.

Since long-time back Government of India (Fig. 7.6) is putting efforts in an order to eradicate anaemia from the country. Still few more attempts are needed. FOGSI has come to the forefront to give fruitful outcome to those attempts and fill up left behind lacunae.

ANAEMIA MUKT BHARAT

A Nation wide Anaemia Mukt Bharat has been planned with evidence-based strategy which include:
1. High political commitment.
2. Target setting.

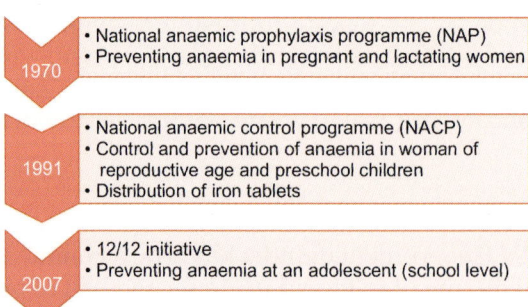

Fig. 7.6: Government initiatives for anaemia prevention

3. Strengthening programme coverage.
4. Strengthening procurement and supply chain management.
5. Intensive behaviour change communication.
6. Robust monitoring and review.

Under this programme following key interventions are included

1. Test and treat malaria in endemic pockets.
2. Use of iron fortified food in public health facilities.
3. Delayed cord clamping after delivery (by 3 minutes).
4. Intensive IEC/BCC for consumption of iron rich food, optimum IYCF and nutrition awareness.
5. Test and treat anaemia in schoolgoing adolescent girls and pregnant women.
6. Iron and folic acid supplementation and deworming.

MANAGEMENT

NICE guidelines recommend that women are screened for anaemia at booking and again at 28 weeks gestation. All women should be given advice regarding diet in pregnancy with details of foods rich in iron along with factors that may promote or inhibit the absorption of iron. This should be backed up with written information. Dietary changes alone are not sufficient to correct an existing iron deficiency in pregnancy and iron supplements are necessary.

ANTENATAL
If at booking Hb <11 gm/dL

Start on a trial of oral iron. The necessary dose is 100–200 mg of elemental iron daily.

Women should be counselled as to how to take oral iron supplementation correctly. This should be on an empty stomach, 1 hour before meals, with a source of vitamin C to maximise absorption. Other medications or antacids, tea or coffee should not be taken at the same time.

Women with a norman Hb but a low MCV should have their ferritin checked and if ferritin is <30 micro/L, oral iron should be commenced.

Repeat Hb levels 3 weeks after commencement of iron therapy (this should fit in with 15–16 week antenatal appointment) and a rise in Hb should be demonstrated. If there is no rise in Hb despite compliance with therapy serum ferritin should be checked and concomitant causes of the anaemia need to be excluded. Referral to consultant obstetrician is required.

If at Booking Hb <9.0 gm/L

Oral iron—200 mg elemental iron in divided doses/day should be commenced and follow up as above. Referral to consultant obstetrician if symptomatic.

If at booking Hb <7.0 gm/L

Send an urgent referral to joint obstetric/haematology clinic to investigate further and make management plan. Do not offer blood transfusion unless symptomatic or currently actively bleeding. Consider total dose IV iron infusion.

200 mg of elemental iron/day (N.B. if 200 mg ferrous sulphate used, need 3–4 tablets/day) if taken correctly will give a rise in Hb of 20 gm/L every 3 weeks.

Once Hb is within the normal range, treatment should be continued for a further three months.

At 28 week: All women should have their Hb re-checked

If at 28 weeks Hb < 10.5 gm/L: Trial of oral iron as above. Re-check Hb in 3 weeks. If no reponse, check serum ferritin and refer to consultant obstetrician to consider total dose iron infusion.

If at 28 weeks Hb <9 gm/L: Start oral iron 200 mg elemental iron in divided doses/day, as above. Consultant obstetrician referral if symptomatic.

If at 28 weeks Hb <7 gm/L: Urgent referral to joint obstetric/haematology clinic to investigate and make management plan. Do not offer blood transfusion unless symptomatic or currently actively bleeding. Consider total dose IV iron infusion.

Gastrointestinal toxicity affects 35–59% of patients and can result in nonadherence to treatment with oral preparations. These effects can be reduced by taking oral iron with food or taking a reduced dose.

Parenteral iron can be considered from the second trimester onwards and during the third trimester for women with confirmed iron deficiency who fail to respond to or are intolerant of oral iron. Intravenous iron is the appropriate treatment for those patients with active inflammatory bowel disease where oral preparations are not tolerated or contraindicated.

MANAGEMENT OF ANAEMIA

In developing countries, it is common to see patients of moderate and severe anemia late in pregnancy. They have had nil or inadequate antenatal care and did not take iron supplements in pregnancy. If the woman presents in mild-trimester or early third trimester, oral iron is started.

Although for prophylaxis the Government of India, Ministry of Health recommends 100 mg of elemental iron with 0.5 mg folic acid, for treatment more than 180 mg of elemental iron per day is required.

Three tablets of ferrous sulphate (available free of cost in most Indian hospitals) per day are required. This may cause increased incidence of side-effects and some recommend 120 mg elemental iron per day, which is more suitable for supplementation rather than treatment. Ferrous ascorbate is the most favourable iron for Indian Diet which have high content of inhibitor for iron absorption 12. One needs to change a brand only when the patient cannot tolerate it. Addition of folic acid, but not vitamin B_{12} helps in improving the results in supervised supplementation. Up to 10% of women may have side effects with oral iron in the form of gastrointestinal symptoms such as nausea, vomiting, constipation, abdominal cramping and diarrhoea which are dose-related. The treatment of choice is to reduce the dose. If this does not work, another preparation (carbonyl) iron or haemoglobin preparations may be better tolerated.

Response to Therapy

Feeling of well-improved look and better appetite. Haematologically, there is reticulocyte response in 5–10 days with a rise in Hb concentration from 0.3–1.0 gm per week and haematocrit subsequently. If there is no significant clinical or haematological improvement within 3 weeks, diagnostic re-evaluation is needed.

Reasons of failure to respond to oral therapy are inaccurate diagnosis (non-iron) deficiency microcytic anaemia, such as thalassaemia, pyridoxine deficiency and lead poisoning), noncompliance, continuous loss of blood through hookworm infestation or bleeding haemorrhoids, coexisting infection, faulty iron absorption and concomitant folate deficiency.

NEWER IRON PREPARATIONS

Iron Amino Acid Chelates

These are conjugates of ferrous or ferric ions with amino acids. Ferrous glycine sulphate is the only iron amino acid chelate available in India. Its main advantage is its relatively high bioavailability in the presence of dietary inhibitors. The chelates prevents iron from binding inhibitors in food or precipitating it as an insoluble complex in the gut.

Sustained release preparations like iron polymaltose complex (IPC) and iron hydroxide polysucrose complex are available. These have nonionic iron in a stable complex. Absorption is not affected by food or milk and these can be given with food. It has better absorption and lesser side effects than ferrous salt.

Carbonyl Iron

It is pure form of elemental iron which has low toxicity and is tolerated in larger does when compared to ferrous salts. Carbonyl iron refer to manufacturing process whereby pentacarbonyl iron is reduced by heating to very fine microsphere of less than 5 microns in diameter which are better absorbed and associated with lesser gastrointestinal side effects. It is available as modified release preparations.

While selecting iron preparations for therapy, it is important to bear in mind that modified release formulations release iron gradually as they pass along the gut hence, a part of the iron is released beyond the most actively absorbing regions of the intestines, that is the first part of the duodenum, thereby reducing overall absorption of iron. Of all the iron preparations ferrous sulphate, ferrous fumarate and ferrous ascorbate are the preferred formulations.

Parenteral Iron Therapy

The rise in Hb concentration is the same, as with oral iron (up to 1 gm per week).
- Indications
- Poor tolerance to oral therapy.
- Poor absorption of iron like in chronic diarrhoea, ulcerative colitis, coeliac disease or inflammatory bowel disease.
- Noncompliance.
- Oral iron is not effective.
- Women near term with severe anaemia.
- Presence of concurrent disease like chronic renal failure when patient is on haemodialysis or being treated with erythropoietin.
- Preparations
- Parenteral iron is available as iron dextran complex (Imferon) which can be given intramuscularly or intravenously.

Iron sorbitol citrate which can only be given, intramuscularly.

Iron sucrose complex each ml has 20 mg of elemental iron.

Iron gluconate is available as sodium ferric gluconate.

Ferric carboxymaltose (FCM) a novel iron complex that consists of a ferric hydroxide core stabilised by a carbohydrate shell, allows for controlled delivery of iron to target tissues.

Administered intravenously, it is effective in the treatment of iron-deficiency anaemia, delivering a replenishment dose of up to 1000 mg of iron during a minimum administration time of </=15 minutes. Results of several randomised trials have shown that intravenously administered ferric carboxymaltose rapidly improves haemoglobin levels and replenishes depleted iron stores in various populations of patients with iron-deficiency anaemia, including those with inflammatory bowel disease, heavy uterine bleeding, postpartum iron-deficiency anaemia or chronic kidney disease.

Ferric carboxymaltose is a macromolecular ferric hydroxide carbohydrate complex, which allows for controlled delivery of iron within the cells of the reticuloendothelial system and subsequent delivery to the iron-binding proteins ferritin and transferrin, with minimal risk of release of large amounts of ionic iron in the serum. Intravenous administration of ferric carboxymaltose results in transient elevations in serum iron, serum ferritin and transferrin saturation, and, ultimately, in the correction of haemoglobin levels and replenishment of depleted iron stores.

The total iron concentration in the serum increased rapidly in a dose-dependent manner after intravenous administration of ferric carboxymaltose. Ferric carboxymaltose is rapidly cleared from the circulation and is distributed primarily to the bone marrow (approximately 80%) and also to the liver and spleen. Repeated weekly administration of ferric carboxymaltose does not result in accumulation of transferrin iron in patients with iron-deficiency anaemia. Intravenously administered ferric carboxymaltose was effective in the treatment of iron deficiency anaemia in several 6- to 12-week, randomised, open-label, controlled, multicentre trials in various patient populations, including those with inflammatory bowel disease, heavy uterine bleeding or postpartum iron-deficiency anaemia, and those with chronic kidney disease not undergoing or undergoing haemodialysis.

In general, improvements in haemoglobin levels were more rapid with ferric carboxymaltose than with ferrous sulfate. Ferric carboxymaltose also replenished depleted iron stores and improved health-related quality-of-life (HR-QOL) in patients with iron-deficiency anaemia. Recipients of ferric carboxymaltose demonstrated improvements from baseline in serum ferritin levels and transferrin saturation, as well as improvements from baseline in HR-QOL assessment scores. Ferric carboxymaltose was at least as effective as ferrous sulphate with regard to endpoints related to serum ferritin levels, transferrin saturation and HR-QOL.

INDICATIONS

Ferric carboxymaltose is an iron replacement product indicated for the treatment of iron deficiency anaemia (IDA) in adult patients who have intolerance to oral iron or have had unsatisfactory response to oral iron, and in adult patients with nondialysis dependent chronic kidney disease.

IMPORTANT SAFETY INFORMATION

Contraindications

Ferric carboxymaltose is contraindicated in patients with hypersensitivity to FCM or any of its inactive components.

Warnings and Precautions

Serious hypersensitivity reactions, including anaphylactic-type reactions, some of which have been life-threatening and fatal, have been reported in patients receiving ferric carboxymaltose. Patients may present with shock, clinically significant hypotension, loss of consciousness, and/or collapse. Monitor patients for signs and symptoms of hypersensitivity during and after administration for at least 30 minutes and until clinically stable following completion of the infusion. Other serious or severe adverse reactions potentially associated with hypersensitivity which included pruritus, rash, urticaria, wheezing, or hypotension were reported.

In clinical studies, hypertension was also reported. Transient elevations in systolic blood pressure, sometimes occurring with facial flushing, dizziness, or nausea were observed in some. These elevations generally occurred immediately after dosing and resolved within 30 minutes.

In the 24 hours following administration of ferric carboxymaltose, laboratory assays may overestimate serum iron and transferrin bound iron by also measuring the iron in ferric carboxymaltose.

Adverse Reactions

The following serious adverse reactions have been most commonly reported from the postmarketing spontaneous reports: urticaria, dyspnoea, pruritus, tachycardia, erythema, pyrexia, chest discomfort, chills, angioedema, back pain, arthralgia, and syncope.

Deficit is Calculated as

Elemental iron needed (mg) = **(Normal Hb – Patient's Hb) × Weight (kg) × 2.21 + 1000**

Here normal haemoglobin is taken as 14% and 2.21 is standard coefficient. To the value calculated by above formula 1000 mg is added for the stores.

Technique of Giving Parental Iron

Intravenous Route

Before giving test dose it is essential to have all the resuscitation equipment and drugs ready. Iron dextran is diluted in normal saline or 5% dextrose and given slowly initially. If there is no reaction, it can be given faster. If the calculated dose is more than 2500 mg, it should be even in 2 doses on two consecutive days. One should look for any reaction in the form of chest pain, rigor, chills, fall in blood pressure, dyspnoea and anaphylactic reaction. For any such reaction, infusion should stopped and anti-histaminic, corticoids and epinephrine given.

The Intramuscular Route

it is more popular and is associated with less side—effects. For giving intramuscular injection it is important to test for hypersensitivity. Full dose of iron can be given daily on alternate buttocks by deep intramuscular injection by Z technique. Oral iron should be stopped before, giving iron sorbitol as it is associated with toxic reaction such as headache, nausea and vomiting.

Disadvantages of Intramuscular Route

Pain, sterile abscess formation nausea, vomiting, headache, fever, lymphadenopathy, allergic reactions and rarely anaphylaxis.

Blood Transfusion

It is required in patients with severe anemia beyond 36 weeks, associated infection, to replenish blood loss due to antepartum or postpartum hemorrhage and in patients not responding to oral or parenteral iron therapy. Packed cells are preferred for transfusion (Fig. 7.7). Blood transfusion can cause transfusion reaction, precipitated preterm labour and, rarely, overloading of the heart.

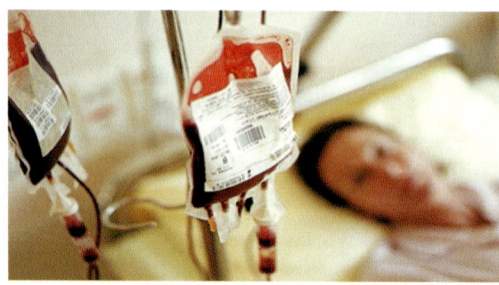

Fig. 7.7: Blood transfusion

General Principles of Blood Transfusion

1. Consent for blood transfutionl
   - Valid consent should be obtained where possible prior to administering a blood transfusion.
   - In an emergency where it is not feasible to get consent, information on blood transfusion should be provided retrospectively.
   - The reason for transfusion and a note of the consent discussion should be documented in the patient's care noted.
2. Requirement for group and screen samples and cross-matching
   - All women should have their blood group and antibody status checked at booking and at 28 weeks.
   - Group and screen samples used for provison of blood in pregnancy should be leass than 3 day old.
3. Blood product specification in pregnancy and puerperium:
   - ABO and Rh compatibility should be done before transfusion.
   - If clinically significant red cell antibodies are present, then blood negative for the relevant antigen should be cross matched before transfusion.
   - CMV seronegative red cell should be provided for elective transfusion during pregnancy.

In sever anamia patient stabilisation is very important. So vigilant monitoring is needed. Blood transfusion should be started under lasix cover. Strict input output charting should be done. Propped up position with O_2 mask and O_2 saturation should me maintained. No fluid overload to be done.

Procedure and Monitoring

Both whole blood and PRBCs contain a small amount of citrate anticoagulant and an additional preservative. Blood collected in citrates phosphate dextrose (CPD) adenine-1 anticoagulant can be stored for up to 35 days and it is essential to start transfusion and return unused blood within 30 minutes of leaving the laboratory. All transfusions should be given and monitored by clinician closely for the first 15 minutes for serious hemolytic reactions, with monitoring of the vital signs every 30 min and infuse for a maximum of 4 hours.

Recombinant Erythropoietin

The stimulation of erythropoiesis with rhEPO is highly promosing alternative to blood transfusion.

Dosage regimen Erythropoietin

Injection erythropoietin can be given subcutaneously or IV 100–150 IU/kg. On day 1, 3 and 5 along with parenteral iron or day 1, 3 and 5 6000 units SC erythropoietin and iron dextran 100 mg deep im daily for 5 day. Dose should be given after subcutaneously sensitivity test. Adrenaline, hydrocortisone and oxygen to be kept ready.

In a simplified way management of anaemia according to the age of gestation varies with the grade of anaemia given in Flow Charts 7.1 to 7.4.

I. At 14–16 Weeks of Gestation

Flow Chart 7.1: Management of anaemia at 14–16 weeks

Deworming with one 400 mg of tablet albendozole after meals at 14–16 weeks

↓

First estimation of blood haemoglobin at 14–16 weeks of gestation by cyanmeth-haemoglobin method using semi-autoanalyser or photocalorimeter

If blood haemoglobin level less than 7 gm/dL	If blood haemoglobin level between 7.1 and 10.9 gm/dL	If blood haemoglobin level than 11 gm/dL
Refer to higher instiutions (CEmONC centres) for blood transfusion and further management	• Therapeutic dose of tablet ferrous sulphate 100 mg of elemental iron 1 BD with 0.5 mg of folic acid • 1 tablet of vitamins B$_{12}$ 15 mcg and vitamin C100 mg/OD to be supplemented	• Prevantive dose of tablet ferrous sulphate 100 mg of elemental iron 1 OD 0.5 mg of folic acid • 1 tablet of vitamin B$_{12}$ 15 mcg and vitamin C 100 mg/OD to be supplemented

II. At 20–24th Weeks of Gestation

Flow Chart 7.2: Management of anaemia at 20–24 weeks

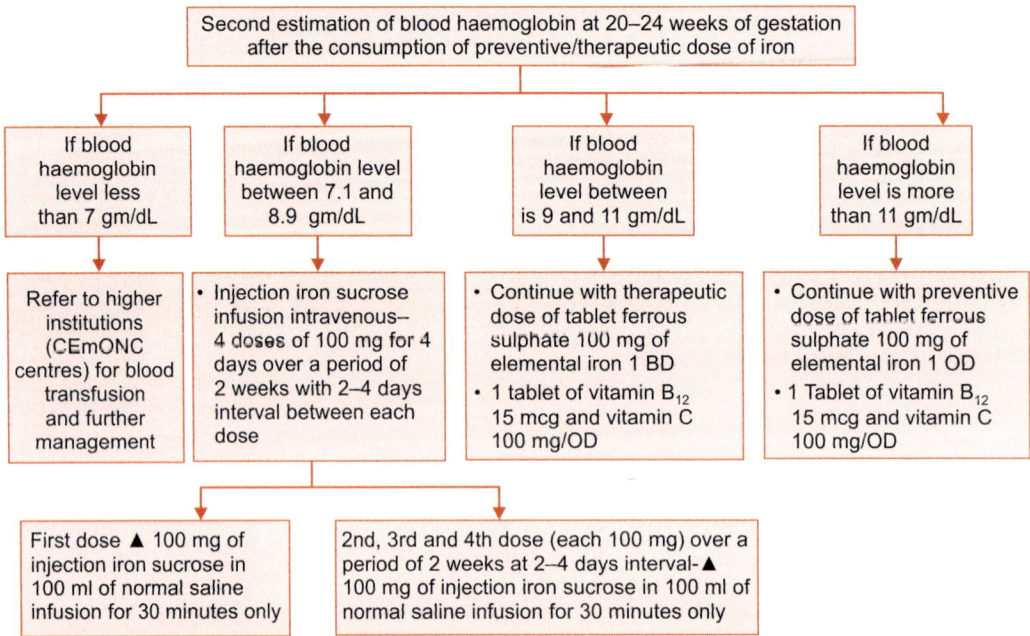

III. At 26–30 Weeks of Gestation

Flow Chart 7.3: Management of anaemia at 26–30 weeks

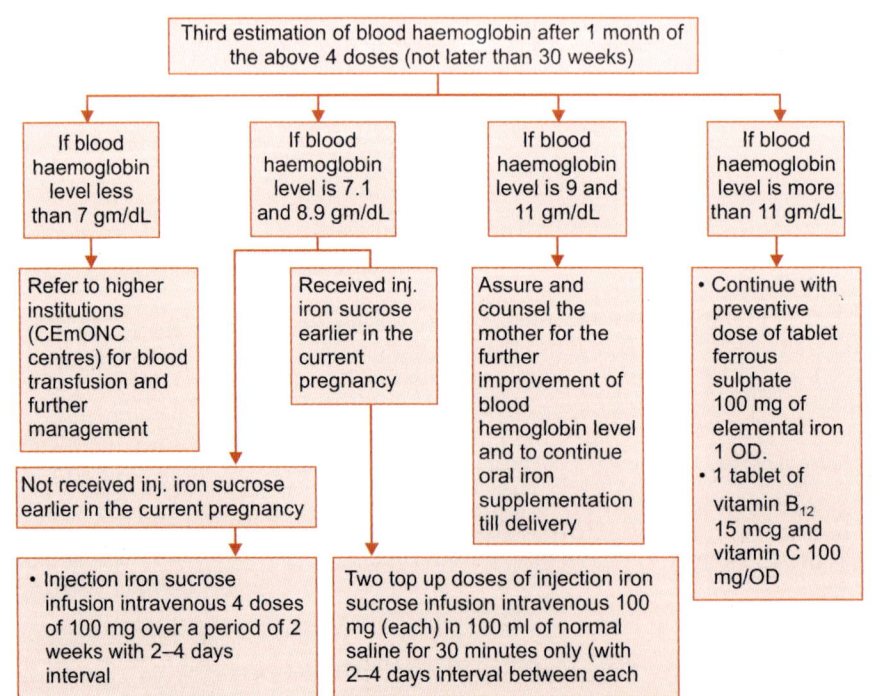

IV. At 30–34 Weeks of Gestation

Flow Chart 7. 4: Management of anaemia at 30–34 weeks

```
                    ┌─────────────────────────────┐
                    │ Estimation of blood haemoglobin at │
                    │    30–34 weeks of gestation        │
                    └─────────────────────────────┘
```

If blood haemoglobin level less than 7 gm/dL	If blood haemoglobin level is 7.1–8.9 gm/dL	If blood haemoglobin level is 9–11 gm/dL	If blood haemoglobin level is more than 9–11 gm/dL
Refer to higher institutions (CEmONC centres) for blood transfusion and further management	Refer to higher institutions (CEmONC centres) for blood transfusion and further management	Assure and counsel the mother for the further improvement of blood haemoglobin level and to continue oral iron supplementation till delivery	• Continue with preventive dose of tablet ferrous sulphate 100 mg of elemental iron 1 OD • 1 tablet of vitamin B_{12} 15 mcg and vitamin C 100 mg/OD

ANTENATAL CARE

The antenatal management is like any other case, but more frequent visits are required. One should be vigilant to detect and manage complications of anaemia, such as heart failure or preterm labour, as early as possible. Foetal monitoring for growth and well-being should be done as these fetuses tend to be small. Prognosis is good if anaemia is detected and treated in time.

MANAGEMENT OF LABOUR IN ANAEMIC PATIENT

In the first stage, the patient should be in a comfortable position. Sedation and pain relief should be given. Oxygen should be kept ready and is given in dyspnoea. In cases of preterm labour, betamimetics and steroids should be given with caution to avoid the risk of pulmonary oedema. Digitalisation may be required in cardiac failure due to severe anaemia. The aim is to deliver the baby vaginally.

Antibiotic prophylaxis is preferred. The second stage is the most stressful, when the patient can go into cardiac failure. A tendency for prolongation of the second stage can be curtailed by forceps. Active management of the third stage should be done except in very severe anaemia for fear of cardiac failure. However, any postpartum haemorrhage must be frenetically treated as these patients tolerate bleeding very poorly. Maternal mortality in severe anaemia can occur in the last trimester, during labour, immediately after delivery and during puerperium due to cardiac failure or pulmonary embolism.

DURING PUERPERIUM

The mother should have adequate rest; iron and folate therapy should be continued for least 3 months. Any infection must be treated. Puerperal sepsis, failing lactation, subinvolution of uterus and thromboembolism are more common in these patients and should be carefully watched for. Maternal mortality in severe anaemia can occur in the last trimester, during labour, immediately after delivery and during puerperium due to cardiac failure or pulmonary embolism.

CONTRACEPTION

The anaemic patient must use an effective method of contraception and should not conceive for at least 2 years giving time for iron stores to recover. Sterilisation is preferred if the family is completed.

If there is no history of menorrhagia, an intrauterine device can be inserted.

Levonorgestrel intrauterine device (Mirena) can be used in presence of menorrhagia for contraception. It reduces blood loss but is expensive. Also progesterone only pill is a good option for contraception. Under the scheme of ANTARA, injection progesterone contraception option is provided free of cost in government hospital.

Barrier methods can be safely given, but their higher failure rate is a disadvantage.

Megaloblastic Anaemia in Pregnancy

INTRODUCTION

The low incidence of megaloblastic anaemia during pregnancy is because of the abundance of both folic acid and vitamin B_{12} (cyanocobalamine) in the vegetarian and nonvegetarian diet. In the developing world the incidence is considerably higher approximately 25% of women with anaemia during pregnancy.

PATHOPHYSIOLOGY

In megaloblastic anaemia (Figs 8.1 and 8.2), DNA replication is affected. There is derangement of red cell maturation with production of abnormal precursors known as megaloblasts which can due to deficiency of folate or vitamin B_{12}.

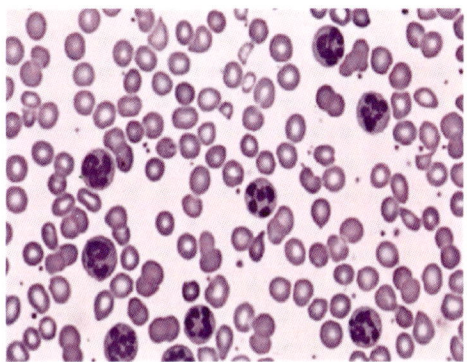

Fig. 8.1: Peripheral blood film of megaloblastic anaemia

Normal anaemia   Megaloblastic anaemia

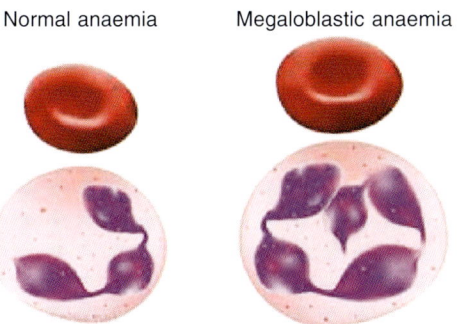

Fig. 8.2: Morphological difference between normal and megaloblastic anaemia

CLINICAL FEATURES

Usually has an insidious onset with gradually progressive symptoms and signs which are usual of anaemia, i.e. weakness, easy fatigability, tiredness, etc. GI symptoms like anorexia, nausea, vomiting, diarrhoea and glossitis more common. Hyperpigmentation of skin and oral mucosa, palpable liver and spleen, petechial rash due to thrombocytopenia may be present and in such case leukaemia and aplastic anaemia should be ruled out.

Nail changes do not occur in megaloblastic anaemia. Occurs more commonly in multiple pregnancies, develops late in pregnancy around 20–28 weeks, develops immediately postpartum or up to fifth month, in OC pill users or in antiepileptic drug users. The cause of megaloblastic anaemia in pregnancy is nearly always due to for the deficiency which leads to folate deficiency and wasting. Hematological symptoms are more marked. If postdelivery haemoglobin level falls rapidly and there is no history of excessive blood loss then suspicion of folic acid deficiency is aroused first.

Folic acid in pregnancy is not always accompanied by significant haematological changes. In the absence of changes, megaloblastic hematopoiesis is suspected when expected response to adequate iron therapy is not achieved. Ultimately diagnosis is dependent on marrow examination and the finding of large erythroblasts and giant abnormally shaped metamyelocytes.

As such vitamin B_{12} deficiency takes years to develop anaemia and its deficiency causes infertility so megaloblastic anaemia due to B_{12} deficiency is very rare in pregnancy. Neurological features are more pronounced and if any autoimmune disease exists in the body with anaemia then suspicion of B_{12} megaloblastic anaemia arises.

DIAGNOSIS

Criteria for Megaloblastic Anaemia

At least two of the following criteria must be present:
   a. More than 4% of neutrophil polymorphs have five or more lobes (Fig. 8.3).
   b. Orthochromatic macrocytes must be present with diameter > 12 mm.
   c. Howell-Jolly (Fig. 8.4) bodies are demonstrated.
   d. Nucleated red cells.
   e. Macropolycytes may be present.

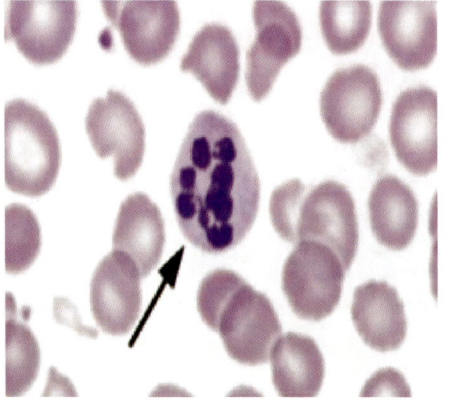

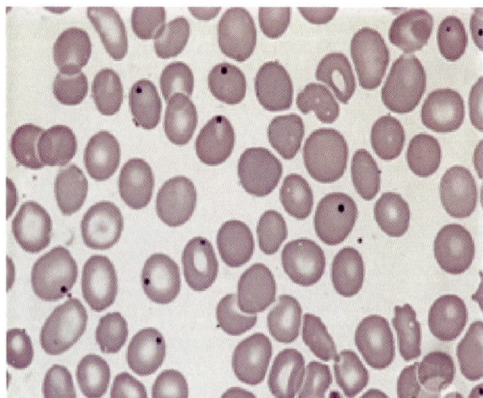

Fig. 8.3: Multilobed neutrophil   **Fig. 8.4:** Howell-Jolly bodies

DIMORPHIC ANAEMIA

This is due to deficiency of both iron and folate with dominance of one in finding of both predominance of that type whose deficiency is more.

FOLATE DEFICIENCY

Effects on Pregnancy

There is increased incidence of abortion, growth retardation, abruption placentae and pre-eclampsia in folate deficiency. Folate supplements during pregnancy have resulted in increased birth weight in cases of malnutrition.

Effects on Foetus

Neural tube defects can be prevented in most cases by periconceptional folic acid in dosage of 0.4 mg/day in low-risk cases and 5 mg/day in high-risk women. Incidence of neural tube defects is very high in India and periconceptional folate supplementation is strongly recommended in all cases. There is some evidence that the incidence of abortion, premature babies, small-for date babies and folate deficiency in the neonates is higher in babies born to mothers with folate deficiency.

Investigations

Laboratory findings consist of a fall in Hb concentration to generally <10 gm/dL, MCV > 96 fI, MCH >.33 pg, and normal MCHC. There is macrocytic anaemia: with hypersegmentation of neutrophils, neutropenia and thrombocytopenia on peripheral blood film. A combination of low serum folate (<3 mg/mL) and red cell folate (<150 ng/mL is diagnostic of folic acid deficiency. Serum iron is usually normal or high. Increased formiminoglutamic acid (FIGLU) in urine following a loading dose of histidine is found in folate deficiency, but the test is rarely done these days. Serum lactic dehydrogenase (LDH) and homocysteine levels are elevated in folate deficiency. The deoxyuridine suppression test helps in differentiating between folate and vitamin B_{12} deficiency. Bone marrow will show a megaloblastic picture, but is rarely required.

Prophylaxis

The WHO recommends a daily folate intake of 800 gm in the antenatal period and 600 gm during lactation. However, 300–500 gm present in most iron preparations is enough for prophylaxis. Pregnant women should eat more green vegetables (e.g. spinach and broccoli) or nonveg (e.g. liver and kidneys). Folate is destroyed by cooking. Even food fortification with folic acid is recommended and is already in use in Western countries.

Treatment

Treatment of established folic acid deficiency by giving 5 mg oral folate per day which should be continued for at least 4 weeks in puerperium.

By 4–7 days of therapy the reticulocyte count is appreciably increased.

VITAMIN B_{12} DEFICIENCY

Pernicious anaemia caused by lack of intrinsic factor resulting in lack of absorption of vitamin B_{12} is rare during pregnancy as it usually causes infertility (Fig. 8.5). Women with gastrectomy and ileal disease and resection can have vitamin B_{12} deficiency. Acquired vitamin B_{12} deficiency causing megaloblastic anaemia is also uncommon, as

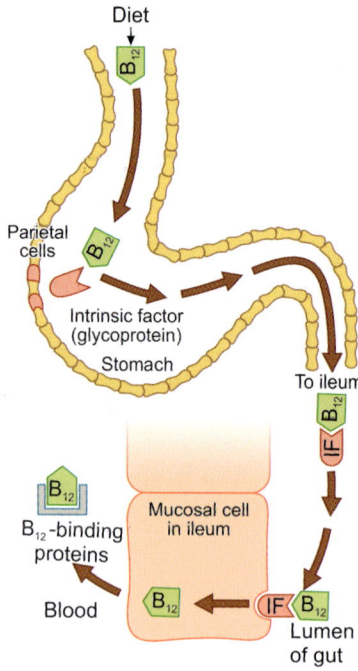

Fig.8.5: Vitamin B_{12} absorption

the daily requirement of vitamin B_{12} is only 3.0 gm during pregnancy which is easily met with a normal diet. Only vegans who do not eat any animal-derived substance may have a deficiency of vitamin B_{12} and they should have their diet supplemented during pregnancy.

Infestations with diphyllobothrium latum in some countries can cause megaloblastic anaemia due to competitive utilisation of ingested vitamin B_{12} by the parasite.

Investigations

Findings are the same as in folate deficiency. Vitamin B_{12} levels are lower in blood (<90 gm/L). Serum methyl malonic acid is elevated in vitamin B_{12} deficiency. Serum homocysteine is elevated in both folate and vitamin B_{12}, deficiency. The deoxyuridine suppression test can differentiate between vitamin B_{12} and folate deficiency. Schilling test is done to diagnose pernicious anaemia.

Treatment

Parenteral cyanocobalamin (250 gm) is given intramuscularly every month.

Nutritional deficiency anaemia during pregnancy continues to be a major health problem in India. To eradicate it certain steps can be taken at individual and community level like education of the women as regards anaemia, its causes and health implication. Imparting nutritional education, with special emphasis on strategies based on locally available foodstuffs to improve the dietary intake of proteins and iron, administration of appropriate iron supplements and ensuring maximum compliance, deworming, treatment of chronic disease like malaria and universal antenatal care to pregnant women will help in combating this serious problem. Long-term policies by government, nongovernment agencies and the community can be directed to formulate effective plans like eradicating anaemia in children and adolescent girls.

Haemolytic Anaemias

Haemolytic anaemias may occur because of erythrocyte defects such as abnormalities of haemoglobin structure metabolic disturbances, or membrane abnormalities. Hence, the classification of haemolytic anaemia as per the aetiology is given here (Table. 9.1). Almost all erythrocyte defects causing haemolysis are hereditary in nature. Haemolysis may also occur due to the presence of substances in the plasma that attack and destroy the erythrocyte such as is the case in autoimmune haemolytic anaemia. A normal red cell lives for about 120 days. This life span is shortened in the case of haemolytic anaemias because of premature destruction of red cells, which may occur extravascularly (i.e. acquired immune haemolytic anaemia or intravascularly (i.e. microangiopathic haemolytic anaemia of pre-eclampsia). Although classifications of anaemias according to the site of haemolysis is important for an adequate interpretation of the laboratory tests for differential diagnosis, in many haemolytic process destruction occurs in both compartments and laboratory tests are ambiguous.

Extravascular haemolysis is the most common haemolytic anaemia. The red cell are destroyed in the reticuloendothelial system, liberating which is converted to bilirubin. An increase in indirect bilirubin is apparent in the patient's serum. The products of bilirubin metabolism, foecal and urinary urobilinogen, also increase. Erythropoiesis

Table 9.1: Classification of haemolytic anaemia

1. Intrensic (intracorpuscular) abnormalities

   A. Hereditary

     i. Membrane abnormalities:

        Membrane skeleton: Spherocytosis, elliptocytosis
                              Membrane lipids: Abetalipoproteinemia

     ii. Enzyme deficiencies: Glycolytic enzymes: Pyruvate kinase, hexokinase;
                              Structurally abnormal globin: Sickle cell anaemia, unstable Hb

   B. Acquired
        Membrane defect: Paroxysmal nocturnal haemoglobinuria

2. Extrinsic (extracorpuscular) abnormalities
   A. Antibody mediated:

       Isohemagglutinins: Transfusion reactions, erythroblastosis foetalis;
                              Autoantibodies: Idiopathic drug associated SLE

   B. Mechanical Trauma: Microangiopathic haemolytic anaemia; TTP, DIC, defective
                              cardiac valves

   C. Infection: Malaria.

increases markedly, and reticulocytosis occurs. Thus, elevated unconjugated bilirubin, increased urinary urobilinogen, and reticulocytosis are the laboratory hallmarks of extravascular haemolysis.

Intravascular and extravascular haemolysis both causes bone marrow response characterised by marked erythroid hyperplasia and reticulocytosis. In some cases the erythroid poiesis is so active that there is passage of immature cells into the bloodstream. Also, in all cases of accelerated red cell destruction, plasma-lactic dehydro (LDH) increases as a consequence of the liberation LDH isoenzyme from the red cells.

The most common form of haemolytic anaemia seen during pregnancy is the intravascular microangiopathic haemolysis, which is a part of the HELLP syndrome.

More infrequently, the obstetrician sees the haemolytic anaemia associated with defects in haemoglobin structure, particularly sickle cell disease (SCD). The World Health Organization (WHO) estimates that globally at least 5% of adults are carriers for a haemoglobin condition: Approximately 2.9% for thalassaemia and 2.3% for sickle cell disease.

MICROANGIOPATHIC HAEMOLYTIC ANAEMIA

Microangiopathic haemolytic anaemia occurs during pregnancy in patients with a severe form of pre-eclampsia, HELLP syndrome. The differential diagnosis in pregnant women can be thrombotic thrombocytopenic purpura (TTP) and haemolytic uremic syndrome.

All of these show fragmented red cell, schistocytes, and burr cells.

Thrombocytopenia is always present. Delivery improves clinical and laboratory in HELLP but not in HUS.

HELLP SYNDROME

It was first described by Weinstein in 1985.

It is the most sever haematological complication of sever pre-eclampsia. In 15% cases, BP of the patient is normal. Most commonly occur in third trimester. Maternal mortality rate is 1% and recurrence rate is 25%.

The acronym HELLP stands for

H = Evidence of haemolysis manifested by
- LDH >600 IU/L
- Elevated bilirubin >1.3 mg/dL
- Low serum haptoglobin
- Abnormal peripheral blood smear—showing schistocytes, burr cells and helmet cell

EL—Elevated liver enzyme AST and ALT >70 IU/L

LP—low platelet count (<1 lakh/mm^3).

Management

If pregnancy is >34 weeks = give prophylactic MgSO$_4$ and immediate delivery. If pregnancy is between 24 and 34 weeks give MgSO$_4$ and corticosteroids (betamethasone 12 mg 2 doses 24 hours apart) and deliver.

Mode of delivery: Vaginal delivery only if cervix is ripe, gestational >32 weeks and FHR is reactive, otherwise caesarean section.

Classification of HELLP

Mississippi Class System

- **Class 1**
  Platelet <50000
- **Class 2**
  Platelet 50000–100000
- **Class 3**
  Platelet 100000–150000
  Haemolysis +
  Elevated Liver enzymes (LDH >600)

Tennessee System

- AST and/or ALT >40
- Platelets <10000
- LDH >600 IU/L
- AST >70

In immune haemolytic anaemia (Fig. 9.1), the patient makes autoantibodies of the immunoglobuli (lgG) type or "warm antibodies" against red cell antigents, causing premature destruction of these cells. In other cases the RBCs are sensitised with both an IgG antibody and complements, usually, C3, more rarely, the RBCs only exhibit complement and no IgG. This abnormality many occur in association with several disease (leukaemia, lymphomas, viral infections) or as a consequence of an immune reaction to certain drugs (penicillin, sulfas, quinidine). The most frequent cause of this abnormality in pregnant women is an autoimmune disorder. On a few occasions, no cause can be discovered and the disorder is named "idiopathic immune haemolytic anaemia."

The diagnosis of immune haemolytic anaemia is made with the direct Coombs' test. In this test, red cells of the patient are mixed with Coombs' antihuman globulin antiserum, and since they are coated with IgG and complement, agglutination occurs immediately.

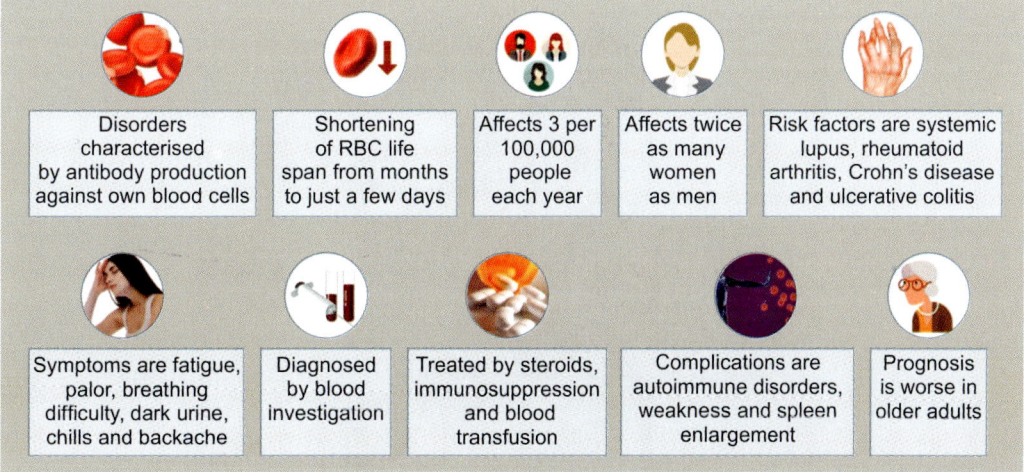

| Disorders characterised by antibody production against own blood cells | Shortening of RBC life span from months to just a few days | Affects 3 per 100,000 people each year | Affects twice as many women as men | Risk factors are systemic lupus, rheumatoid arthritis, Crohn's disease and ulcerative colitis |

| Symptoms are fatigue, palor, breathing difficulty, dark urine, chills and backache | Diagnosed by blood investigation | Treated by steroids, immunosuppression and blood transfusion | Complications are autoimmune disorders, weakness and spleen enlargement | Prognosis is worse in older adults |

Fig. 9.1: Autoimmune haemolytic anaemia

Haemoglobinopathies

SICKLE CELL DISEASE (SCD)

It is the most common haemoglobinopathy encountered during pregnancy because of the severity of the applications associated with this condition. Sickle cell disease in pregnancy is a high-risk and management should be given for optimal maternal and neonatal outcome.

SCD is an autosomal recessive (Fig. 10.2) condition caused by the substitution of a valine for glutamine in position 6 in the beta-globin chain of the haemoglobin molecule, resulting in the proteins on of sickle cell haemoglobin (Fig. 10.1), or HbSS. The condition affects 0.2% of the African- American population of USA. In India it is common in the tribal population of central India. The disease is characterised by chronic haemolytic anaemia and by the occurrence of acute, life-threatening occlusive crisis. It is associated with increased maternal and perinatal morbidity and mortality.

Sickle-Cell Trait

The heterozygous inheritance of the gene for haemoglobin S results in sickle-cell trait, or AS haemoglobin. The trait is not associated with increased abortion, perinatal mortality, low birth weight, or pregnancy-induced hypertension. Sickle cell trait therefore should not be considered a deterrent to pregnancy on the basis of increased maternal risks. In SCD when HbS is oxygenated, its solubility is similar to that of normal haemoglobin (HbSS) but in the deoxy form solubility decreases and in a

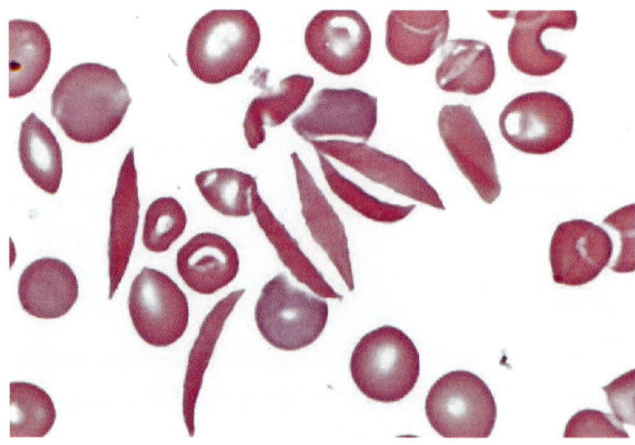

Fig. 10.1: Peripheral blood film of sickle cell disease

How the trait is passed on

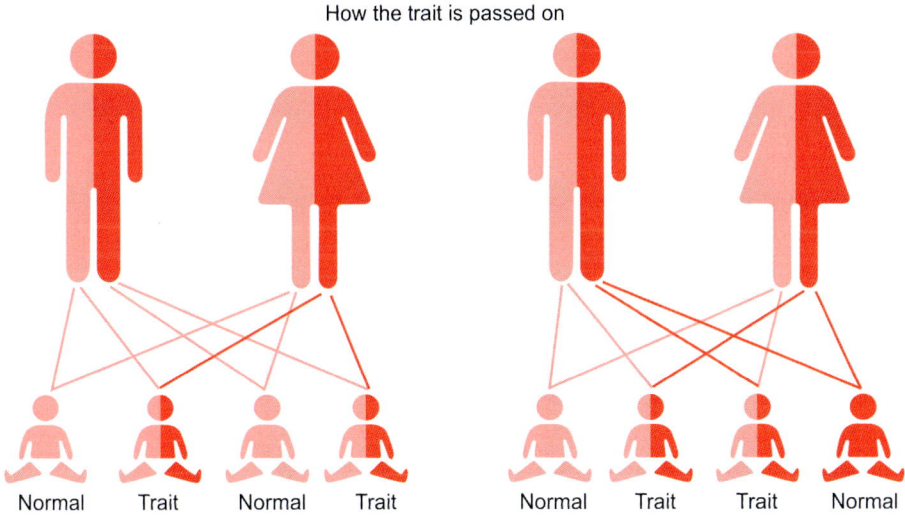

| Normal | Trait | Normal | Trait | | Normal | Trait | Trait | Normal |

Fig 10.2: Inheritance of sickle cell disease

reduced oxygen environment the HbSS will polymerise into long tube like fibres, which causes morphological changes characterised by sickling of the erythrocytes. The abnormal erythrocytes are removed and destroyed in the reticuloendothelial system, resulting in chronic extravascular haemolysis. HbF inhibits the polymerisation of HbSS and patients with elevated levels of HbF have milder forms of the disease. In certain situations such as increased deoxygenation, acidosis, fever, dehydration, prolonged capillary transit time. Concentration of corpuscular haemoglobin and clusters of sickle cells occlude the microvasculature, producing ischaemic infarction and severe inflammatory reactions that clinically translate into a painful sickle cell crisis. Around 14.2% of all pregnancies in patients with SCD end with the delivery of stillborn infants and neonatal morality is approximately 84.5 per 100 live births.

The frequency of infants with birth weights less than 2500 gm in patients with SCD is increased.

Acute chest syndrome are most common cause of mortality in patients with SCD. It is characterised by chest pain, respiratory distress with tachypnoea, coughing and wheezing, fever, decreased oxygen saturation.

Infection is a frequent-cause of sickle cell crisis but diagnosis is difficult because many of the signs and symptom of a vaso-occlusive crisis are similar to those of infection. Fever, leukocytosis, elevated bilirubin, and LDH are also components of crises. Relief of the severe pain, reduction in HbSS concentration and to increase oxygen supply to the tissues are the tenets of management. Treatment usually involves pain management, oxygen, antibiotics, incentive spirometry, bronchodilators, and most case transfusion therapy.

Prenatal Diagnosis

Women with sickle cell trait should always undergo preconception counselling.

The male partner should also be examined to determine whether or not he carries the trait. The father is a carrier, there is a 25% chance that the infant will be homozygous and have SCD. Early prenatal genetic diagnosis is important because it will allow the possibility of pregnancy termination. Early prenatal diagnosis is possible with the use of polymerase chain reaction (PCR).

Amniocentesis or Chorionic Villous Sampling.

Antepartum Care

- Close observation.
- Folic acid supplementation.
- Identify sickle cell crisis: Adequate hydration to be maintained.
- Screening and treatment for bacteriuria.
- Assessment of fetal health: Weekly antepartum foetal surveillance beginning at 32 to 34 weeks with serial ultrasonography to monitor foetal growth and amniotic fluid.
- Prophylactic transfusions in women with a history of multiple vaso-occlusive episodes and poor obstetrical outcomes.

Patients with SCD do not require iron supplemental and during pregnancy unless laboratory evidence of iron deficiency is obtained. In contrast, they need adequate folic acid supplementation to compensate for the increased consumption of folate secondary to the active process of cell replication that takes place in their bone marrow.

Labour and Delivery

- Adequate analgesia.
  Epidural analgesia: Ideal.
- Compatible blood should be available.
- If haematocrit is less than 20% packed erythrocyte transfusions are administered
- Prevent circulatory overload and pulmonary oedema from ventricular failure.

Postpartum Management

- Early ambulation to prevent venous thrombosis.
- Adequate hydration.
- Analgesic drugs should be given for pain relief.
- Cord blood should be sent for electrophoresis.

Contraception

Progesterone-based contraception like Depot medroxy progesteron acetate is safe and has beneficial effect of decreasing sickling due to stabilisation of erythrocyte membrane. Barrier method is widely used but rate of failure is high. Permanent method is advised on completion of family.

THALASSAEMIA IN PREGNANCY

There are many point mutations in the globin gene that may cause beta thalassaemia minor, and this, explains the clinical variability of the condition (Fig. 10.3). In this condition HbA2 is increased more than 3.5 %.

HbF is usually increased to more than 2%. The anaemia is microcytic and hypochromic, and there is basophilic stippling of the erythrocytes.

The haemoglobin levels range from 8 to 10 gm/dL. The diagnosis is frequently missed, and the patients are repeatedly treated with large doses of oral, and in some instances parenteral, iron without therapeutic response. This is dangerous because they may develop hepatic and cardiac haemosiderosis secondary to iron overload.

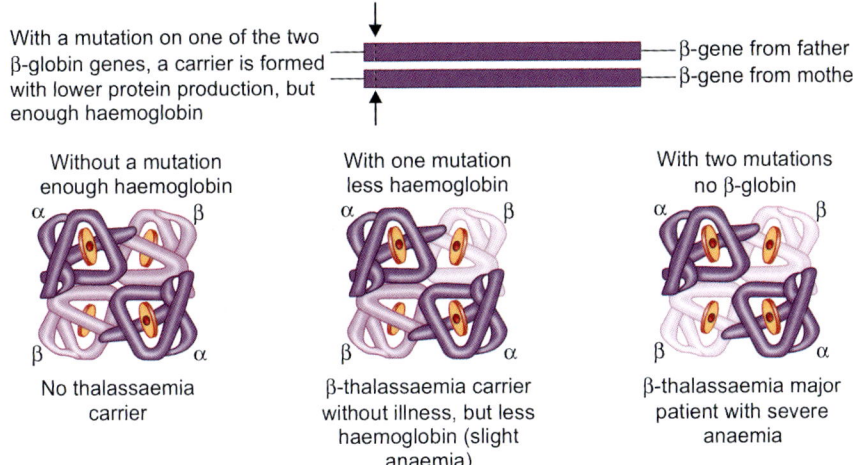

With a mutation on one of the two β-globin genes, a carrier is formed with lower protein production, but enough haemoglobin

β-gene from father
β-gene from mother

Without a mutation enough haemoglobin	With one mutation less haemoglobin	With two mutations no β-globin
α β	α β	α β
β α	β α	β α
No thalassaemia carrier	β-thalassaemia carrier without illness, but less haemoglobin (slight anaemia)	β-thalassaemia major patient with severe anaemia

Fig. 10.3: Pathophysiology of thalassaemia

The diagnosis of beta thalassaemia minor should be suspected when the MCV is 75 fl or less and the RBC is greater than 4.5–5.0 million cells/L. If doubts remain, measurements of serum ferritin and serum iron will clarify the dilemma.

Pregnant partner microcytic, hypochromic anaemia who does not respond to oral iron by an elevation of her haemoglobin concentration after 4 weeks of treatment. Patients with beta thalassaemia minor characteristically, show haemoglobin A2 (HbA2) concentrations greater than 3.5% and normal or increased serum iron concentrations. In 90% of the cases the HbA2 level is above 5%. Approximately 50% of women with beta thalassaemia minor will exhibit a haemoglobin F concentration greater than 2%.

BETA THALASSAEMIA MAJOR

This is a serious disease where both the beta chains are defective. The neonate with this condition is healthy at birth but become severely anaemic as the HbF falls with failure to thrive. Such a child needs blood transfusion to survive and there is problem of iron overloading. In the past most children with beta thalassaemia major used to die, but are now reaching reproductive age group with blood transfusion and chelation therapy with deferoxamine. Such women are usually sterile with shorten lifespan.

However, some women had successful pregnancy outcome under intensive maternal and fetal surveillance by an experienced team of haematologist and obstetrician. They need cardiac assessment for myocardial function. There anaemia should be treated with blood transfusion, folic acid supplementation required. Iron supplementation is contraindicated.

Naked Eye Single Tube Red Cell Osmotic Fragility Test (NESTROFT)

The principle of NESTROFT is based on the limit of hypotonicity which the red cell can withstand. In this procedure 2 ml of 0.36% buffered saline is taken in a test tube, 20 ml of whole blood is added to it, and is allowed to stand at room temperature. After 20 minutes reading is taken on a NESTROFT stand on which a thin black line is marked. If the line is visible through the solution, the test is considered as negative and if line is not visible it is considered as positive. Positive test is due to the reduced osmotic fragility of red cells (Fig. 10.4).

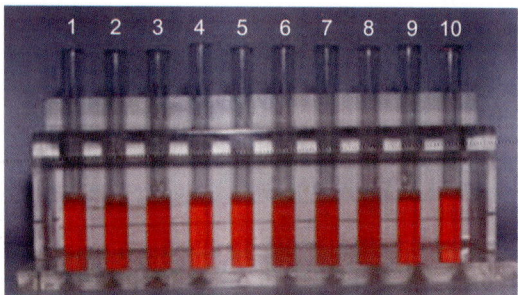

Fig. 10.4: NESTROFT stand showing positive and negative samples in different tubes. Tubes from L to R: Tubes 1–3 and 6–8 are positive samples where black line is not visible through the solution, tubes 4–5 and 9–10 negative samples where black line is visible through the solution

Aplastic Anaemia

INTRODUCTION

Although aplastic anaemia was first recognised by Ehrlich in 1888, the pathogenesis of aplastic anaemia has remained elusive. Prevalence of aplastic anemia in pregnancy is rare. Aplastic anaemia is a subtype of anaemia characterised by pancytopenia and a hypocellular bone marrow (Fig. 11.1). This condition can be due to chemicals, drugs, infections, irradiation, leukaemia, and inherited disorders. The treatment involves immunosuppressive therapy with antithymocyte globulin and cyclosporine and bone marrow transplantation.

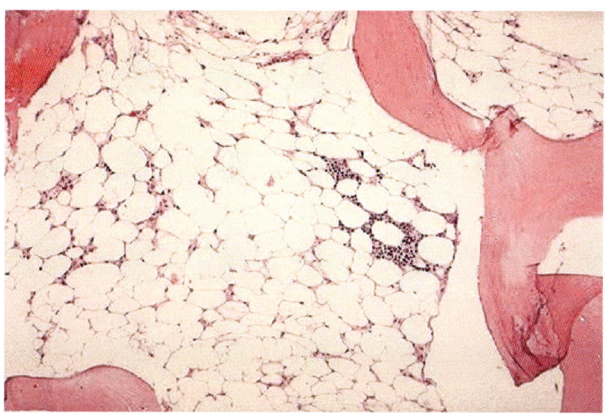

Fig. 11.1: Bone marrow smear of aplastic anaemia

There is universal agreement that pregnancy complicated by aplastic anaemia is a serious condition. There is risk to the mother mainly in the form of haemorrhage and sepsis. The foetus may suffer from growth restriction and even intrauterine death. Haemorrhage and sepsis are responsible for more than 90% of maternal mortality.

Most of the foetal complications are due to maternal anaemia. All along with these, maternal infections may lead to the development of chorioamnionitis and resultant preterm labour and birth.

In the literature, foetal thrombocytopenia, placentomegaly, and severe oligohydramnios have also been reported. We here present two cases of pregnancy complicated by aplastic anaemia, which were seen within a span of 1 year at our hospital. This high incidence is because the hospital is a tertiary care referral unit with good haematology and blood bank support.

Aplastic anaemia is a serious haematological disorder characterised by pancytopenia (Fig. 11.2), bone marrow hypocellularity, and even absence of underlying malignant or myeloproliferative disease.

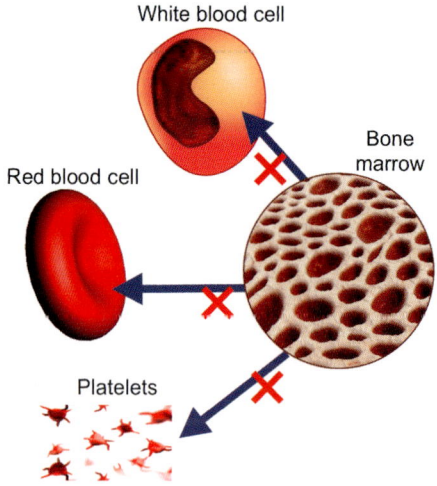

Fig. 11.2: Cells affected in aplastic anaemia

Aplastic anaemia is known to increase the antenatal complications in pregnancy. On the literature review, the rate of preterm birth was 12.1%, intrauterine death was 16.7%, stillbirth was 15.1%, and spontaneous miscarriage was 16.7% among pregnant women with the diagnosis of aplastic anaemia. Postpartum haemorrhage is an important complication among patients with the diagnosis of aplastic anaemia due to decreased platelet count. In cases of aplastic anaemia, vaginal birth is preferred, and caesarean section is performed only for obstetric indications. In general, treatment for aplastic anaemia includes withdrawal from offending drugs, supportive care, and some form of definitive therapy. Bone marrow transplantation (BMT) has been reported to be the most effective treatment, with a 5-year survival of 56–89%. However, BMT is contraindicated during pregnancy because it requires high-doses of immunosuppressive agents or radiation therapy, which would be toxic to the foetus. Although case reports have suggested a promising result with antithymocyte immunoglobulin (ATGAM) or cyclosporine therapy during pregnancy, there is currently little agreement on the universal use of these therapies. The role of androgens is not clear. Androgen treatment may cause the virilisation of female fetuses. The efficacy of corticosteroids or granulocyte colony-stimulating factor is also equivocal. The current evidence does not favour the routine use of any drug therapy in the treatment of pregnancy-associated aplastic anaemia. Earlier case reports have suggested termination as an alternative approach.

Cyclosporine (300 mg/day) and granulocyte macrophage colony-stimulating factor (450 mg intravenous weekly) have been used in severe aplastic anaemia after 20 weeks of pregnancy though data regarding their use in pregnancy with aplastic anaemia is limited. However, experience from pregnancy following organ transplant shows that cyclosporine is apparently not teratogenic. Though it is excreted in milk, foetal growth and development were found to be normal. Perhaps the most important part of treatment of aplastic anaemia is supportive therapy. Supportive therapy in the form of repeated blood and platelet transfusions are given to keep haemoglobin above 10.5 gm/dL and platelet count at above 20×10^9/L.

Platelet

INTRODUCTION

Platelets or thrombocytes (Fig. 12.1) are the formed elements of blood. Platelets are small colourless, non-nucleated and moderately refractive bodies. These formed elements of blood are considered to be the fragments of cytoplasm.

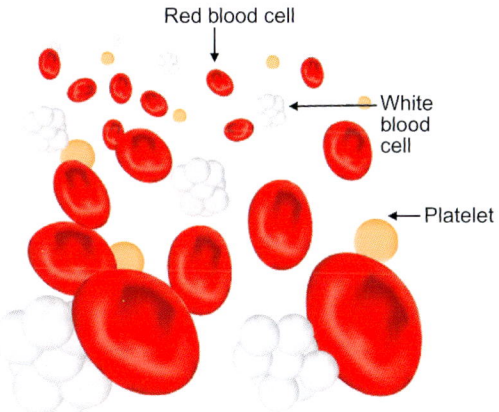

Red blood cell

White blood cell

Platelet

Fig. 12.1: Platelets

Size of Platelets

Diameter: 2.5 (2 to 4)

Volume: 7.5 cu (7 to 8 cu).

Shape of Platelets

Normally, platelets are of several shapes, viz. Spherical or rod-shaped and become oval or disk-shaped when inactivated. Sometimes, the platelets have dumbbell shape, comma shape, cigar shape or any other unusual shape. Inactivated platelets are without processes or filopodia and the activated platelets develop processes or filopodia.

STRUCTURE AND COMPOSITION

Platelet is constituted by (Fig. 12.2):

1. Cell membrane or surface membrane
2. Microtubules
3. Cytoplasm.

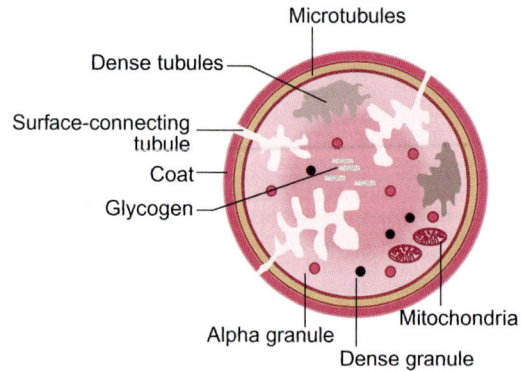

Fig. 12.2: Morphology of platelet

Cell Membrane

Cell membrane of platelet is 6 nm thick. Extensive invagination of cell membrane forms an open canalicular system. This canalicular system is a delicate tunnel system through which the platelet granules extrude their contents. Cell membrane of platelet contains lipids in the form of phospholipids, cholesterol and glycolipids, carbohydrates as glycocalyx and glycoproteins and proteins. Of these substances, glycoproteins and phospholipids are functionally important.

Glycoproteins

Glycoproteins prevent the adherence of platelets to normal endothelium, but accelerate the adherence of platelets to collagen and damaged endothelium in ruptured blood vessels. Glycoproteins also form the receptors for adenosine diphosphate (ADP) and thrombin.

Phospholipids

Phospholipids accelerate the clotting reactions. The phospholipids form the precursors of thromboxane A_2 and other prostaglandin-related substances.

Microtubules

Microtubules form a ring around cytoplasm below the cell membrane. Microtubules are made up of polymerised proteins called tubulin. These tubules provide structural support for the inactivated platelets to maintain the disklike shape.

Cytoplasm

Cytoplasm of platelets contains the cellular organelles, Golgi apparatus, endoplasmic reticulum, mitochondria, microtubule, microvessels, filaments and granules. Cytoplasm also contains some chemical substances such as proteins, enzymes, hormonal substances, etc.

Proteins

1. Contractile proteins

   i. *Actin and myosin:* Contractile proteins, which are responsible for contraction of platelets.
   ii. *Thrombosthenin:* Third contractile protein, which is responsible for clot retraction.

2. *von* **Willebrand factor:** Responsible for adherence of platelets and regulation of plasma level of factor VIII.

3. **Fibrin-stabilising factor:** A clotting factor.

4. **Platelet-derived growth factor (PDGF):** Responsible for repair of damaged blood vessels and wound healing. It is a potent mytogen (chemical agent that promotes mitosis) for smooth muscle fibres of blood vessels.

5. **Platelet-activating factor (PAF):** Causes aggregation of platelets during the injury of blood vessels, resulting in prevention of excess loss of blood.

6. **Vitronectin (serum spreading factor):** Promotes adhesion of platelets and spreading of tissue cells in culture.

7. **Thrombospondin:** Inhibits angiogenesis (formation of new blood vessels from pre-existing vessels).

Enzymes
1. Adensosine triphosphatase (ATPase).
2. Enzymes necessary for synthesis of prostaglandins.

Hormonal Substances
1. Adrenaline
2. 5-hydroxytryptamine (5-HT; serotonin)
3. Histamine.

Other Chemical Substances
1. Glycogen.
2. Substances like blood group antigens.
3. Inorganic substances such as calcium, copper, magnesium and iron.

Platelet Granules
Granules present in cytoplasm of platelets are of two types:
1. Alpha granules.
2. Dense granules.

Alpha Granules
Alpha granules contain
1. Clotting factors—fibrinogen, V and XIII.
2. Platelet-derived growth factor.
3. Vascular endothelial growth factor (VEGF).
4. Basic fibroblast growth factor (FGF).
5. Endostatin.
6. Thrombospondin.

Dense Granules
Dense granules contain
1. Nucleotides.
2. Serotonin.
3. Phospholipid.

4. Calcium.
5. Lysosomes.

NORMAL COUNT AND VARIATIONS

Normal platelet count is 2,50,000/cmm of blood. It ranges between 2,00,000 and 4,00,000/cmm of blood.

PHYSIOLOGICAL VARIATIONS

1. *Age*: Platelets are less in infants (1,50,000 to 2,00,000/cmm) and reaches normal level at third month after birth.
2. *Sex*: There is no difference in the platelet count between males and females. In females, it is reduced during menstruation.
3. *High altitude*: Platelet count increases.
4. *After meals*: After taking food, the platelet count increases.

PROPERTIES OF PLATELETS

Platelets have three important properties (three 'A's):
1. Adhesiveness
2. Aggregation
3. Agglutination.

Adhesiveness

Adhesiveness is the property of sticking to a rough surface. During injury of blood vessel, endothelium is damaged and the subendothelial collagen is exposed. While coming in contact with collagen, platelets are activated and adhere to collagen. Adhesion of platelets involves interaction between von Willebrand factor secreted by damaged endothelium and a receptor protein called glycoprotein Ib situated on the surface of platelet membrane. Other factors which accelerate adhesiveness are collagen, thrombin, ADP, thromboxane A_2, calcium ions, P-selectin and vitronectin.

Aggregation (Grouping of Platelets)

Aggregation is the grouping of platelets. Adhesion is followed by activation of more number of platelets by During activation, the platelets change their shape with elongation of long filamentous pseudopodia which are called processes or filopodia . Filopodia help the platelets aggregate together. Activation and aggregation of platelets is accelerated by ADP, thromboxane A_2 and platelet-activating factor (PTA: cytokine secreted by neutrophils and monocytes).

Agglutination

Agglutination is the clumping together of platelets. Aggregated platelets are agglutinated by the actions of some platelet agglutinins and platelet-activating factor.

FUNCTIONS OF PLATELETS

Normally, platelets are inactive. They execute their actions only when activated. Activated platelets release many substances. This process is known as platelet release reaction. Functions of platelets are carried out by these substances. Functions of platelets are:

Role in Blood Clotting

Platelets are responsible for the formation of intrinsic prothrombin activator. This substance is responsible for the onset of blood clotting.

Role in Clot Retraction

In the blood clot, blood cells including platelets are entrapped in between the fibrin threads. Cytoplasm of platelets contains the contractile proteins, namely actin, myosin and thrombosthenin, which are responsible for clot retraction.

Role in Prevention of Blood Loss (Haemostasis)

Platelets accelerate the haemostasis by three ways (Fig. 12.3):

   i. Platelets secrete 5-HT, which causes the constricttion of blood vessels.

  ii. Due to the adhesive property, the platelets seal the damage in blood vessels like capillaries.

 iii. By formation of temporary plug, the platelets seal the damage in blood vessels.

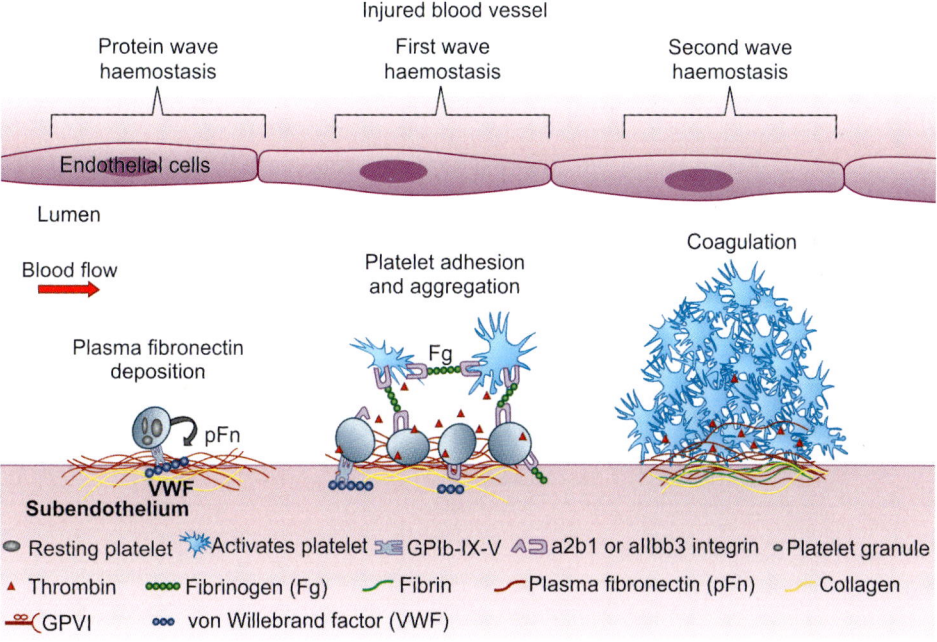

Fig. 12.3: Mechanism of haemostasis

ROLE IN REPAIR OF RUPTURED BLOOD VESSEL

Platelet-derived growth factor (PDGF) formed in cytoplasm of platelets is useful for the repair of the endothelium and other structures of the ruptured blood vessels. Substances released from dense granules of platelets.

Coagulation Cascade and Platelet Disorder in Pregnancy

In the 1960s two groups proposed a model of coagulation as a sequential series of steps in which activation of one clotting factor leads to the activation of another, finally leading to a burst of thrombin generation. Each clotting factor was thought to exist as a proenzyme, which was converted to an active enzyme by proteolysis.

The original "cascade" or "waterfall" models were subsequently modified to include the observation that some procoagulants are cofactors that do not possess enzymatic activity. In addition, the clotting sequences were divided into so-called extrinsic and intrinsic systems (Fig. 13.1). Both pathways activate factor X, which, in complex with its cofactor Va, converts prothrombin to thrombin. A phosphatidylserine-containing phospholipids surface and calcium are essential for the activity of the coagulation complexes. We currently assess the components of the extrinsic pathway clinically with the prothrombin time (PT) test and the components of the intrinsic pathway with the activated partial thromboplastin time (APTT) tes.

The cascade concept of coagulation was extremely valuable, but many people recognised that the intrinsic and extrinsic systems could not operate *in vivo* as independent and redundant pathways as it is explained theoretically. It was clear that

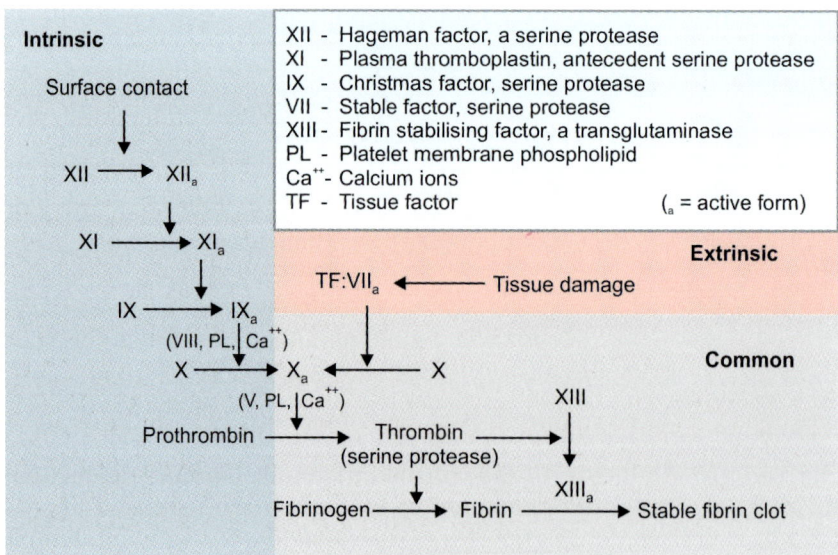

Fig. 13.1: Coagulation cascade

even though deficiencies of each of the factors in the intrinsic pathway could produce equally long APTT values, they have dramatically different risks of haemorrhage. For example, deficiencies of factor XII are not associated with significant haemorrhage, deficiencies of factor XI might or might not be associated with haemorrhage, and deficiencies of factors VIII and IX are consistently associated with haemorrhage.

Cells are important participants in the coagulation process. Of course, normal haemostasis is not possible in the absence of platelets. Also, TF (tissue factor) is an integral membrane protein and thus its activity is normally associated with cells.

Initiation and amplification of coagulation: The role of the tissue-factor-bearing cell.

The goal of haemostasis is to produce a platelet and fibrin plug to seal a site of injury in the blood vessel wall. Haemostasis is initiated when TF-bearing cells are exposed to blood at a site of injury. TF is a transmembrane protein that acts as a receptor and cofactor for factor VII. Once bound to TF, zymogen factor VII is rapidly activated through mechanisms not yet completely understood; they may involve autoactivation and activation by noncoagulation proteases.

The resulting factor VIIa/TF complex catalyzes two reactions: the activation of factor X and the activation of factor IX.

The factor Xa and IXa formed on TF-bearing cells have distinct and separate functions in initiating blood coagulation. Factor Xa interacts with its cofactor Va to form prothrombinase complexes and generates a small amount of thrombin (factor IIa) on TF-bearing cells.

By contrast, the factor IXa activated by FVIIa/TF does not act on the TF-bearing cell and does not play a significant role in the initiation phase of coagulation. If an injury has occurred and platelets have adhered near the TF-bearing cells, the factor IXa can diffuse to the surface of nearby activated platelets. It can then bind to a platelet surface receptor , interact with its cofactor, factor VIIIa, and activate factor X directly on the platelet surface.

Most coagulation factors can leave the vasculature; their activation peptides are found in the lymph. Therefore, it is likely that most (extravascular) TF is bound to factor VIIa even in the absence of an injury, and that low levels of factor IXa, factor Xa, and thrombin are produced on TF-bearing cells at all times. This process is kept separated from key components of haemostasis by an intact vessel wall, however. The very large components of the coagulation process are platelets and factor VIII bound to multimeric von Willebrand factor (VWF). These components normally enter the extravascular space only when an injury ruptures the vessel wall. Platelets and VIII-VWF can then leave the vascular space and adhere to collagen and other matrix components at the site of injury.

Binding of platelets to collagen or via VWF leads to a degree of platelet activation, but the coagulation process is most effectively initiated when enough thrombin is generated on or near the TF-bearing cells to fully activate platelets, as well as factors V, VIII, and XI. Although this amount of thrombin may not be sufficient to clot fibrinogen, it is sufficient to amplify the initial procoagulant signal and set the stage for a subsequent burst of thrombin generation on platelet surfaces. The small amounts of factor Va required for prothrombinase assembly on TF-bearing cells are activated by factor Xa or by noncoagulation proteases produced by the cells. The small amounts of thrombin generated on TF-bearing cells are responsible for activating platelets, factor V, factor VIII (and dissociating it from VWF), and factor XI. The activity of the factor Xa formed by the factor VIIa/TF complex is restricted to the TF-bearing cell, because any factor Xa that dissociates from the cell surface is rapidly inhibited by tissue factor pathway inhibitor (TFPI) or antithrombin (AT) in the fluid phase. In contrast to factor Xa, factor IXa can diffuse to adjacent platelet surfaces because it is not inhibited by TFPI and is inhibited only slowly by AT.

Propagation of thrombin generation and formation of the fibrin clot: The role of platelets play a major role in localising clotting reactions to the site of injury because they adhere and aggregate at sites where TF is also exposed. They provide the primary surface for generation of the burst of thrombin needed for effective haemostasis during the propagation phase of coagulation. Platelet localisation and activation are mediated by VWF, thrombin, platelet receptors, and vessel wall components such as collagen.

Once platelets are activated, the cofactors Va and VIIIa rapidly localise to the platelet surface. As mentioned above, the factor IXa formed by the factor VIIa/TF complex can diffuse through the fluid phase and can also bind to the surface of activated platelets. Likewise, factor XI also binds to platelet surfaces and is activated by the small amount of thrombin produced during initiation of coagulation, thus bypassing the need for factor XIIa. The platelet-bound factor XIa can activate more factor IX to IXa. The specific receptors on activated platelets that bind factor IXa also promote formation of active factor IXa/VIIIa (tenase) complexes. Once the platelet "tenase" complex is assembled, factor X from the plasma is activated to factor Xa on the platelet surface. Factor Xa then associates with factor Va to generate a burst of thrombin sufficient to clot fibrinogen and stabilise the initial platelet plug in a fibrin meshwork. Factor XIII, activated by thrombin, crosslinks fibrin and further stabilises the haemostatic plug. Thrombin also activates the thrombin-activated fibrinolysis inhibitor (TAFI), which helps prevent lysis of the fibrin clot.

PLATELET DISORDER IN PREGNANCY

Thrombocytopenia

Thrombocytopenia is low platelet count, if present during pregnancy can jeopardise the maternal and foetal outcome. Thrombocytopenia affects 6–15% of pregnancies. The increasing report of thrombocytopenia is also be attributed to better antenatal check-ups and performance of investigation like complete blood count (CBC). It is defined as platelet count less than $150 \times 10^9/L$. Pregnancy does per se alter platelet level to a great extent but slight changes takes place, which are more pronounced towards term.

Causes

1. Gestational thrombocytopenia.
2. Immune thrombocytopenic purpura.
3. Severe pre-eclampsia.
4. Systemic lupus erythematosus.
5. HELLP.
6. Disseminated intravascular coagulation.
7. Thrombotic thrombocytopenic purpura.
8. Haemolytic uraemic syndrome.
9. Drug-induced thrombocytopenia.

Thrombocytosis

Both pregnancy and essential thrombocytosis (ET) are hypercoagulable states. When they coexist, the complication risk for both mother and foetus is magnified, but which complications, how magnified, and for whom are still unresolved questions.

Management

Treating women with ET during pregnancy is challenging because patients are at increased risk for first trimester spontaneous abortions, thrombotic and obstetric complications, whereas cytoreductive therapy might have harmful effects on the foetus. It has been recommended cytoreductive agents to be avoided, particularly in the first trimester and none is licensed for use in pregnancy.

Women who have an unplanned pregnancy on HU should stop treatment. Anagrelide is also contraindicated during pregnancy. Pregnant women who are candidates for platelet lowering therapy according to general guidelines of ET treatment should receive IFNa which seems to be the safest option for all patients while trying conceiving. Treatment with peg-IFN is more attractive due to the longer half-life and the similar efficacy in controlling platelet count; nevertheless, there is limited data concerning safety profile.

Treatment with low dose aspirin might positively influence the outcome of pregnancy due to reduced probability of placental infarctions. LMWH is reasonable to be considered in women with history of thromboembolic events in the past and high-risk pregnancies for thrombotic potential (for instance immobilisation, twin-pregnancies, high body weight of the patient) or presence of antiphosphilipid syndrome. Inherited thrombophilia like presence of heterozygous F-Leiden mutation, in the absence of positive thrombotic family history, is not a definite indication for anticoagulation in all trimesters. However, special attention should be made during third trimester when LMWH should be initiated until six weeks postpartum.

Gestational Thrombocytopenia

Gestational thrombocytopenia (GT; defined as a platelet count below 150000) occurs in 4.4–11.6% of pregnancies, accounting for about 75% of all cases of thrombocytopenia in pregnancy. Thrombocytopenia is more prevalent in twin and triplet gestations. Platelet counts in many women show a gradual downward trajectory beginning in the second trimester, which is most likely from haemodilution related to an increase in plasma volume during pregnancy and possibly increased platelet clearance as mean platelet volumes, platelet volume distribution width, and platelet derived cyclooxygenase products rise.

A subset of women with GT develop a more significant decline in platelet count and a reduction in antithrombin III, suggesting a discrete pathogenesis that lies on a continuum with the haemolysis, elevated liver enzymes, low platelets (HELLP) syndrome and acute fatty liver of pregnancy (AFLP) and that may be associated with a higher risk of recurrence in subsequent pregnancies.

From the perspective of the haematology consultant, practical points to be emphasised include:

1. A platelet count of 150000/L is; 2 standard deviations below the mean at term.
2. GT does not become apparent before the mid-second trimester.
3. Only 1–5% of women develop platelet counts below 150000/L and few have counts below 150000/L, but counts below 150000/L have been attributed to GT on rare occasions and only when other possible aetiologies have been ruled out.
4. There are no biomarkers to provide an affirmative diagnosis, which might preclude distinction from mild ITP, the onset of pre-eclampsia/HELLP or other diagnoses of exclusion.
5. GT does not intrinsically reflect or affect the health of the mother and foetal thrombocytopenia is uncommon (2%) and mild.
6. GT does not respond to IV immune globulin (IVIG) or corticosteroids, which has been tried when thrombocytopenia is so severe as to compromise epidural anaesthesia or delivery.
7. If thrombocytopenia does not resolve within 1–2 months of delivery, the diagnosis of ITP or HT may become evident only in hindsight.

Management

- Antenatal.
- Monitor platelet count every 4–6 weekly.
- All the pathological causes to be excluded.

During Labour/Delivery

Traumatic vaginal delivery should be avoided to minimise maternal risk of haematoma formation.

Caesarean section should be done in case of obstetric indication.

Epidural anaesthesia is safe in case platelet count is more than 80000.

If count is less than 80000, cord sample should be taken at the time of delivery and on first as well as fourth day.

Postdelivery

After delivery verify that counts have returned to normal.

Immune Thrombocytopenic Purpura

Incidence and diagnosis ITP "i.e. Immune thrombocytopenic purpura or also called as idiopathic thrombocytopenic purpura" occurs in 1 in 1000 to 10000 pregnancies. Although ITP accounts for only; 3% of all cases of thrombocytopenia during pregnancy, it is the most common cause of a platelet count below 50000/L detected in the first and second trimesters. Platelet counts may fall during gestation, and at least 15–35% of mothers require treatment even prior to management of labour and delivery. Maternal and neonatal outcomes are generally favourable. Therefore, ITP is not a contraindication to pregnancy per se. However, in unusually severe or refractory cases or for women reliant on potentially teratogenic medications, deferring pregnancy may be indicated.

There is no laboratory test to distinguish ITP from GT or some of the other causes of maternal thrombocytopenia. Therefore, the diagnosis of ITP is based on a personal history of bleeding, a low platelet count prior to pregnancy, and/or a family history that excludes HT; the diagnosis of ITP is made by excluding other disorders when possible or may be made only retroactively based on response to ITP-directed therapy. A few women lack an antecedent (pregestational) history. ITP should be suspected when an otherwise healthy mother (bleeding excepted) who is taking no medications and has no relevant family or gestational history of concern presents with a platelet count below 50000–80000/L in the first or second trimester and has a peripheral blood smear notable only for thrombocytopenia without unusually small or giant platelets.

Management treatment (Tables 15.1 and 15.2) is initiated for bleeding when the platelet count falls below 20000–30000/L, and for procedures and delivery. Data indicate an increased risk of bleeding if platelet count is below 20000–30000/L for a vaginal delivery or below 50000/L for a caesarean section. Haematomas following neuraxial anaesthesia are exceedingly rare in patients with stable ITP and a platelet count above 50000/L with no concomitant coagulopathy or exposure to an antithrombotic agent.

Platelet counts should be measured more frequently starting at 32–34 weeks and repeated weekly in unstable patients. This generally allows enough time for a change in therapy to improve platelet counts and reduce the risk of bleeding in advance of a planned or unplanned caesarean section or neuraxial anaesthesia without the urgent need for platelet transfusions.

e-Aminocaproic acid is a safe and effective adjunct that should be considered before and after delivery in women with severe ITP and other causes of thrombocytopenia that place a woman at high-risk for bleeding.

Care should be coordinated with an experienced obstetrician and neonatologist to the extent possible. For initial short-term treatment, e.g. in anticipation of delivery,

Table 15.1: Medical management of ITP in pregnancy—ASH and BCSH guidelines

	ASH	BCSH
Treatment indications	• Platelets <10,000/L • Platelets 10,000–30,000/L in 2nd or 3rd trimester bleeding	• Platelets <20,000 / L, unless deliver imminent
IVIg	• Initial treatment: 3rd trimester and platelets <10,000/L • Initial treatment: patelets 10,000–30,000/L and bleeding • After steroid failure: platelets <10,000/L • After steroid failure: platelets 10,000–30,000/L and bleeding • After steroid failure: 3rd trimester, platelets 10,000–30,000/L, asymptomatic	• Oral corticosteroids and IVIg have similar responses as in nonpregnant state
Splenectomy	• 2nd trimester, platelets <10,000/L, bleeding	• If essential, in the second trimester • Laparoscopic approach advantageous
Safe platelet count for delivery	• 50,000/L	• Vaginal delivery: 50,000/L • Caesarean section: 80.000/L • Epidural anaesthesia: 80,000/L

Table 15.2: Management of delivery in patients with pregnancy associated ITP–ASH and BCSH guidelines

	ASH	BCSH
Cordocentesis or foetal scalp sampling	• Not necessarily required • Unnecessary in women without known ITP	• Not recommended
Caesarean section	• In selected circumstances • Appropriate if foetal platelet count is <20,000/L • Not indicated if foetal platelet count unknown • Not indicated if maternal platelet count >50,000/L	• Obstetric indications only
Safe platelet count if delivery	• Vaginal delivery: 50,000/L • Caesarean section: 50,000/L	• Vaginal delivery: 50,000/L • Caesarean section: 80.000/L • Epidural anaesthesia: 80,000/L

daily oral prednisone may be favoured over pulse dexamethasone because there is less concern about placental transfer.

IVIg is used if corticosteroid therapy fails or if its use is limited by maternal intolerance. There is limited published experience with IV immunoglobulin G (IgG) anti-RhD, which crosses the placenta and coats foetal erythrocytes.

Splenectomy has been performed safely in the second trimester, but is rarely required. Persistent exposure to high-dose corticosteroids in the first trimester is associated with a small increased risk of cleft palate and exposure throughout gestation may increase the risk of preterm birth and gestational diabetes. Therefore, greater reliance is often placed on periodic administration of IVIg than would be typical in the management of nonpregnant patients.

There is little evidence on which to base treatment of women refractory to a combination of corticosteroids and IVIg.

Human recombinant thrombopoietin (not currently available in the United States) has been used with success in 1 pilot study, 20 and there are anecdotal reports involving the use of thrombopoietin receptor agonists such as romiplostim in the weeks prior to delivery.

It is difficult to define the risk to the foetus of individual immunosuppressive agents due to the lack of disease-specific and disease-severity controls. The effects on pregnancy outcome and on the foetus of other medications used to treat ITP are either: unknown (thrombopoietin receptor agonists), tolerable/associated with some risks but used for other indications in the setting of pregnancy (azathioprine, cyclosporine, and cyclophosphamide), or known to be teratogenic and not used in pregnancy (mycophenylate; danazol). Dapsone has been associated with a risk of haemolytic anaemia and hyperbilirubinemia in the newborn. Rituximab is not known to be teratogenic but has been associated with prolonged B-cell lymphocytopenia and the need to delay vaccination in neonates exposed *in utero*; therefore, when clinically appropriate, rituximab should not generally be used within at least 6 months of planned conception. ITP does not prevent thrombosis; therefore, thromboprophylaxis and anticoagulation should be managed according to standard protocols. Until evidence-based guidelines are available, our preference is to maintain the platelet count above 20000–30000/L for prophylactic intensity anticoagulation and above 40000–50000/L for therapeutic intensity anticoagulation in the absence of complicating features.

Disseminated Intravascular Coagulation

Disseminated intravascular coagulation (DIC) is a syndrome of abnormal coagulation and fibrinolysis. Consumption coagulopathy is a disorder marked by reductions in blood concentrations of platelets due to exhaustion of the coagulation factors in the peripheral blood as a result of DIC.

It occurs in response to certain obstetric complications that are listed below.

AETIOLOGY

- Eclampsia or pre-eclampsia.
- Postpartum haemorrhage.
- Sepsis.
- Abruptio placentae.
- Missed septic abortion.
- Sickle cell crisis.
- Ruptured uterus T.
- Trophoblastic disease (choriocarcinoma).
- Hypovolaemic shock or massive blood transfusion.
- Amniotic fluid embolism.
- Intrauterine death.

In obstetrics, DIC is always secondary to another health condition of the woman.

The method of activation of the clotting system may be:

Release of thromboplastins into the maternal circulation from placental and decidual tissue: This may happen suddenly in cases of abruptio placentae, amniotic fluid embolism, ruptured uterus, etc. and much more insidiously in the case of intrauterine death and missed abortion. In pregnancies complicated by abruptio placentae with enough severity to cause foetal death, DIC will supervene in about 25% of women. In women with intrauterine death or missed abortion, approximately 25% will develop DIC 5 to 6 weeks after foetal demise, with laboratory changes that, in some cases, become apparent from the start. With early ultrasound diagnosis and the use of prostaglandins to produce cervical changes and facilitate evacuation of the uterus, DIC caused by intrauterine death is likely to decrease. Injury to endothelial cells exposing the underlying collagen to the plasma and coagulation factors: This may be the initiating factor in some cases of eclampsia or pre-eclampsia and sepsis. Red blood cell or platelet injury leading to release of phospholipids: This may occur in blood transfusion reactions.

PATHOPHYSIOLOGY

Normal haemostasis is a dynamic balance between coagulation, leading to fibrin formation, and the fibrinolytic system, which acts to dispose of fibrin when its haemostatic function has been fulfilled. In DIC, there is excessive and widespread coagulation due to the release of thromboplastins into the maternal circulation. This leads to consumption and depletion of the coagulation factors resulting in a haemorrhagic diathesis. In response to the widespread coagulation and fibrin deposition in the microvasculature, the fibrinolytic system is secondarily activated. This involves conversion of plasminogen to plasmin, which breaks down fibrin to form fibrin degradation products (FDP). FDP have anticoagulant properties, inhibiting both platelet function and the action of thrombin, thus further aggravating the coagulation defect.

Haemorrhage diathesis is the main problem in most cases, but in some cases, widespread microvascular thrombosis can cause organ ischaemia and infarction. This may be an accessory factor in the genesis of renal cortical necrosis in cases with severe abruptio placentae.

CLINICAL FEATURES

1. The main symptoms and signs are those of the obstetric complications causing the DIC.
2. Haemorrhagic manifestations may be relatively subtle with bruising, purpuric rash, epistaxis, and venipuncture oozing, or more dramatic with profuse bleeding from operative sites and postpartum haemorrhage.
3. Thrombotic sequelae rarely present in acute DIC as they are overshadowed by the haemorrhagic diathesis. The most common thrombotic manifestations are renal, hepatic, and pulmonary dysfunction.

DIAGNOSIS

Awareness of the obstetric conditions that may trigger DIC and the presenting clinical features is essential. Often the urgency of the situation and the lack of sophisticated laboratory facilities prevent definitive haematological tests. Interpretation of test results may also be difficult because the DIC process is so dynamic that results, when available, will often not reflect the current status of the woman. In severe cases of DIC, virtually all of the tests of coagulation and fibrinolysis will be abnormal, but in milder cases, the results are variable (Table 16.1).

Bedside Clot (Observation) Test

This is the most available and simplest test. An abnormal test indicates gross abnormality of the coagulation system. It is done by taking 5 ml of blood in a glass tube (or syringe), holding it in your fist to keep it warm, while inverting or tipping the tube three or four times and observing the following:

- Clotting time is prolonged if it takes greater than 7–8 minutes for a clot to form.
- Clot consolidation and retraction: The clot should be able to withstand inversion of the tube after 30 minutes and should not lyse or breakdown within 1 hour. The clot should occupy at least half of the total blood sample.

Table 16.1: Criteria for diagnosis of DIC

	ISTH criteria	JMHW criteria	JAAM criteria
Underlying clinical condition predisposing to DIC	Essential	1 point	Essential
Clinical symptoms	Not used	Bleeding = 1 point Organ failure = 1 point	SIRS score ≥3 = 1 point
Platelet count 10^9/L	50–100 1 point	80–120 1 point	80–120 or > 30% reduction = 1 point
	<50 = 2 points	50–80 = 2 points	<80 or >50 reduction = 2 points
		<50 = 3 points	
Fibrin-related marker	Moderate increase = 2 points	FDP 10–20 µg/mL = 1 point	FDP 10–25 µg/mL = 1 point
	Marked increase = 3 points	FDP 20–40 µg/mL = 2 points FDP >40 µg/mL = 3 points	FDP >25 µg/mL = 3 points
Fibrinogen	<1 = 1 point	1–1.5 = 1 point <1 = 2 points	Not used
PT	Prolongation 3–6 sec = 1 point	PT ratio 1.25–1.67 = 1 point	PT ratio ≥1.2 = 1 point
	Prolongation >6 sec = 2 points	PT ratio >1.67 = 2 points	
DIC diagnosis	≥5 points	≥7 points	≥4 points

Where laboratory facilities are available, additional testing will reveal the following results:

- Platelet levels (platelet count) may be low or progressively fall.
- Partial thromboplastin time (PTT) is variable and may only be prolonged later in the process when the clotting factors are severely depleted.
- Prothrombin time (PT) or International Normalized Ratio (INR) will become prolonged.
- Thrombin time (TT) is usually prolonged.
- Fibrinogen levels (fibrinogen assay) are normally increased in pregnancy to 400–650 mg/dL. In DIC, the level falls but may be in the normal nonpregnant range. With severe DIC, the fibrinogen levels usually fall below 150 mg/dL.
- FDP: Levels of 80/mL confirm a DIC diagnosis. However, these elevated levels will remain for 24–48 hours after the DIC has been controlled.
- A blood film or blood smear may show abnormally shaped (helmet or tear-shaped) and fragmented red blood cells (schistocytes). These are formed by the alteration of normal red blood cells as they are forced through the fibrin mesh in the obstructed capillary bed.

MANAGEMENT AND TREATMENT

In most obstetric situations, DIC develops rapidly. Treatment must be prompt. Often, both time and facilities do not permit the luxury of thoroughly delineating the deficient clotting mechanisms. The process and progress of DIC is so dynamic that laboratory results may not reflect the current situation. This does not mean that one should not try and follow the laboratory aspects of the coagulopathy and enlist the aid of a haematologist if available. It does mean, however, that even without detailed haematological evaluation, one must have a rational management plan that will cover most of the problems encountered in this potentially disastrous complication.

Treat the Initiating Cause

Until the obstetric complication leading to the DIC occurs, most women who develop coagulopathy are healthy young women, although some may already suffer from anaemia or malnourishment. These women have a great ability to recover rapidly and completely once the initiating cause is removed. In most cases, this entails emptying the uterus.

Maintain Organ Perfusion

In women, in whom the cause, or result, of DIC is haemorrhage, maintaining organ perfusion is the most urgent and important principle to follow. This is best accomplished by:
- Rapid infusion of Ringer's lactate or normal saline.
- Rapid replacement with whole blood (fresh blood is best, if available, because of its higher concentration of clotting factors and functional platelets).

In most women, swift treatment of the initiating cause and maintenance of organ perfusion are all that is required for successful treatment. Once the cause of DIC has been removed, the liver will replenish adequate levels of most coagulation factors within 24 hours. The platelet count may take 5 to 6 days to return to normal, but will probably reach adequate levels for haemostasis within 24 hours.

Where Additional Resources are Available

Where resources, in addition to those already mentioned, are available:
- Administer oxygen by face mask or by endotracheal intubation and intermittent positive pressure ventilation, if necessary, to achieve satisfactory arterial oxygenation.
- Monitor the above by a central venous pressure line if possible.
- Monitor the urinary output. Aim to keep the urinary output at least 30–60 mL/hour.
- Monitor the complete blood count. Aim to keep the haematocrit >30%.

Replacement of Procoagulants

The use of these is best guided by a haematologist. Knowing that the initiating cause of DIC is being treated, it is logical to think that critical and low procoagulant levels should be replaced to facilitate haemostasis and the adage adding fuel to the fire does not apply.
- Fresh frozen plasma replaces most clotting factors and has the least risk of transmitting hepatitis. As a working rule, give 1 unit after the initial 4 to 6 units of whole blood and thereafter 1 unit for every 2 units of whole blood required.
- Cryoprecipitates may be necessary if fibrinogen levels are low.
- Platelets can be transfused in severe cases of thrombocytopenia. One unit of platelets can raise the number of platelets to about 5,000 to 10,000.
- Inhibition of the disseminated intravascular coagulation and fibrinolysis.

The use of heparin has been advised as a method of blocking DIC. It is recommended for chronic DIC like intrauterine death syndrome. Chronic DIC is considered a less severe form of DIC. It produces no or only mild symptoms, such as bleeding from the skin or mouth. It is not recommended if the woman is bleeding profusely.

Epsilon aminocaproic acid inhibits the conversion of plasminogen to plasmin; its use has been suggested as a means to counteract secondary fibrinolysis. It is not recommended in these cases.

Their use is to a large extent theoretical, and wide practical experience with them is lacking. Their potential for worsening the haemorrhagic diathesis is very real. An exception may possibly be justified in the woman with intrauterine death who is not bleeding, but has strong laboratory evidence of DIC and coagulation factor deficiency. In these rare cases, under the guidance of an expert haematologist, one may consider an intravenous infusion of 1,000 units of heparin per hour until the clotting factors are restored to normal levels. Steps can then be taken to empty the uterus.

Walking Blood Bank

Obtaining blood in a developing country is a problem because blood banks are rarely available. This is complicated if some of the adult population has HIV or other blood-borne infections. When an obstetric emergency requires a transfusion, relatives are asked to donate their blood. It is important that bottles and tubing required for drawing and transfusing the blood be available. This does not allow for testing the blood for HIV, hepatitis, or other blood-borne diseases. To make safer blood available, the concept of a walking blood bank has been developed. Potential donors are identified and their blood is grouped. They are then called to give a blood donation once a woman's blood group has been determined. Blood compatibility is assured before the blood is drawn. Potential donors can be tested for HIV and hepatitis.

Haematological Malignancy During Pregnancy

Cancer is diagnosed in approximately 0.1% of pregnant women and its prevalence is expected to rise in developed countries because of the increase in the average age at pregnancy. Haematologic malignancies complicating pregnancy are uncommon, but a delay in diagnosis or treatment can mean the difference between life and death. It is the responsibility of the obstetrician to maintain a high index of suspicion when patients present with unexplained lymphadenopathy or protracted constitutional symptoms. Due to the relative rarity of this situation, there is often no consensus on the optimal management of the patient. Management of a haematological malignancy during pregnancy can be a challenging process. Management of these patients requires a multifaceted team from the oncology, paediatrics, and obstetrics services. With most haematologic cancers now requiring multi agent chemotherapy for optimal survival. Infants exposed *in utero* to chemotherapy, however, seem to suffer no long-term detrimental consequences.

Hodgkin's Lymphomas (HL)

HL is more frequent than NHL in pregnant women. Near about 3% of HL patients are diagnosed during pregnancy. As compared to nonpregnant female HL in pregnant women is usually diagnosed at the same disease stage. Moreover, the outcome in women who were diagnosed in pregnancy, does not appear to be worse compared to nonpregnant patients.

Non-Hodgkin's Lymphomas (NHL)

Pregnancy itself may obscure symptoms and clinical findings of lymphoma. Pregnant women with aggressive lymphomas (Burkitt or Burkitt-like) may present with an advanced stage disease due to delay in diagnosis. When adequate chemotherapy regimens are administered, survival rates of pregnant patients with NHL are similar to those of nonpregnant controls.

Reproductive organs are commonly get involved in pregnancy-associated NHL than in nonpregnant patients diagnosed with a similar lymphoma subtype. It may because of either due to the increased blood flow to reproductive organs during gestation or due to expression of gestational hormone receptors.

Acute Leukemia

Acute leukemia can affect both the pregnant woman and the foetus. Problems associated with this condition include maternal severe pancytopenia associated with bleeding and infections, disseminated intravascular coagulation, which may significantly complicate the treatment of the mother and the delivery, placental effects of leukaemic cells such as decreased blood flow, and decreased exchange of oxygen and nutrients. The diagnosis of acute leukaemia during pregnancy is a devastating event for the patient and family, necessitating prompt, difficult decisions in the setting of a rapidly evolving condition that is potentially life-threatening. Thankfully, such occurrences are rare with a prevalence of approximately 1 in 100000 pregnancies.

Acute leukaemia is a medical emergency which can result in complications of thrombosis, haemorrhage and leukostasis also increases the risk of abortion, perinatal mortality, intrauterine growth retardation and preterm delivery.

Multiple Myeloma

The median age at diagnosis of MM is 70 years; accordingly, there are few case reports of MM during pregnancy. Disease features such as low back pain and anaemia are frequent during normal pregnancies, which may cause delay in diagnosis.

Chronic Myeloid Leukaemia (CML)

Chronic myeloid leukaemia (CML), a relatively slow-growing tumour, can present with severe leukostasis and vascular complications, adversely affecting maternal and foetal outcomes.

Myeloproliferative Neoplasms

The most common philadelphia chromosome negative MPN are polycythemia vera, essential thrombocytosis (ET) and myelofibrosis. Accordingly, most cases of MPN during pregnancy are those of essential thrombocytosis, and less frequently of polycythemia vera. These diseases are typically seen in older adults; however, 20% of ET patients and 15% of polycythemia vera patients are younger than 40 years at diagnosis.

It is associated with an elevated risk of thrombosis and with pregnancy risk increases. Pregnant women with MPN are at an increased risk of developing thrombosis and other gestational complications like recurrent abortion, premature delivery, foetal growth restriction or loss and pre-eclampsia.

Treatment

Treatment of cancer during pregnancy remains a challenge because the common treatment modalities may produce detrimental effects on the foetus, including foetal demise, congenital malformations, carcinogenesis, intrauterine growth restriction and mental retardation. The decision to employ chemotherapy or radiotherapy during pregnancy should be weighed against the pregnancy stage and the effect of delaying treatment on maternal survival.

Chemotherapy

Physiological changes during pregnancy affect drug pharmacokinetic. Most cytotoxic agents are known to cross the human placenta and reach the foetus circulation. The first trimester is the most critical period for chemotherapeutic drug exposure, as implantation (weeks 1 to 2) and embryogenesis proceed (weeks 3 to 8) during this period. Manifestations of drug toxicity are spontaneous abortions and malformations. It is recommended that folate antagonists (e.g. methotrexate) be avoided during first and second trimesters of pregnancy due to a high-risk of congenital malformations.

CHEMOTHERAPEUTIC AGENT AND ASSOCIATED RISK

Cytarabine—a higher risk for limb deformities.

Anthracycline—a higher risk for eye and limb deformities.

Anthracyclines—higher risk for a development of heart failure in adult patient.

The use of chemotherapy during the first trimester of pregnancy is considered dangerous to the foetus. If chemotherapy is required in the first trimester, pregnancy termination is to be recommended. When termination of pregnancy is not acceptable to the patient, a single agent followed by multi agent therapy at the end of the first trimester can be considered.

Toxic effects of chemotherapy on the foetus during the second and third trimesters are low birth weight, intrauterine growth restriction, premature birth and stillbirth. The CNS continues to evolve throughout the gestation period and therefore, impaired functional development, intellectual disability and diminished learning capability may occur.

Chemotherapy could be administered during the second and third trimesters. However, extreme caution is warranted and detailed discussion with the patient of associated risks should always take place. Delivery should be postponed for 2–3 weeks following treatment to allow bone marrow recovery and foetal drug elimination via the placenta.

Chemotherapeutic agents vary in their concentration in breast milk so most authorities recommend avoiding breastfeeding until at least 2 weeks following the completion of chemotherapy.

Biological Therapy

Rituximab

Based on the available limited data, it is considered that the benefits of rituximab treatment of life-threatening haematologic malignancies during the second and third trimesters of pregnancy may outweigh its risks. Data on teratogenicity are limited and, so the use of rituximab cannot be widely recommended during the first trimester.

Imatinib

Imatinib is the standard of care for nonpregnant patients with CML. Second-generation tyrosine kinase inhibitors are teratogenic. Due cessation of imatinib most of patients developed rapid disease recurrence but achieved remission with reinstitution of imatinib.

Radiotherapy

Foetus exposure to radiation during the first trimester is associated with risk of teratogenesis which is directly proportional to dose of exposure and an increased risk of childhood malignancy. Radiotherapy given in the second and third trimesters is associated with an increased risk for the development of leukaemia and solid tumours within the first decade of life and increased risk of neurodevelopmental impairment.

Radiation should be avoided during pregnancy, apart from highly selected cases such as stage I-II lymphoma confined to the neck or axillary lymph nodes, in the absence of alternative therapies. An expert radio-oncologist must evaluate foetal radiation exposure in each case.

Supportive treatment

Antiemetics

There has been no association found between therapy with metoclopramide, antihistamines or ondansetron-based antiemetics and congenital malformations in either animal models or humans.

Growth Factors

Experience regarding the treatment of chemotherapy-induced cytopenias with granulocyte colony-stimulating factor and erythropoietin is limited; however, no teratogenic effects have been reported to date.

Anti-infective Agents

Aminoglycosides and metronidazole do not appear to be teratogenic. Quinolones and tetracyclines should be avoided during pregnancy. Sulfonamides should be avoided when possible. The safety of penicillins and cephalosporins for the foetus is well-established. The systemic antifungal drug most widely used in pregnancy is amphotericin B.

Disease-specific Therapy

Hodgkin's Lymphomas (HL)

Adriamycin, bleomycin, vinblastine and dacarbazine (ABVD), the most common chemotherapy regimen for HL, is not recommended during the first trimester as data regarding its safety during pregnancy are limited.

Patients with advanced HL diagnosed at an early pregnancy stage should start chemotherapy immediately and pregnancy termination should be strongly recommended in these cases.

Patients with early-stage HL diagnosed in the first trimester can be closely followed-up for signs of disease progression and start chemotherapy in the second trimester.

Patients with HL diagnosed in the second or third trimester can be treated with ABVD, based on limited available data.

Non-Hodgkin's Lymphomas (NHL)

Indolent lymphoma

Treatment may be postponed until delivery or at least until the second trimester. If there is an indication for therapy during the first trimester, single-agent rituximab should be carefully considered. Rituximab plus cyclophosphamide, doxorubicin, vincristine, prednisone (R-CHOP) or rituximab plus cyclophosphamide, vincristine and prednisone (R-CVP) regimens can be used for the management of these lymphomas during the second or third trimester.

Aggressive lymphoma (including large B-cell lymphomas, mantle cell lymphoma and mature T-cell neoplasms):

In the majority of patients with aggressive lymphoma prompt administration of intensive combination chemotherapy, i.e. rituximab plus cyclophosphamide, doxorubicin, vincristine, prednisone (R-CHOP) is required. Information on the safety of its use during the first trimester is limited. Very few studies have suggested safe use of R-CHOP regime during pregnancy.

Highly aggressive lymphoma (including precursor [B or T] lymphoblastic leukaemia/lymphoma and Burkitt's lymphoma):

Due fulminant nature of the disease and rapid progression demands prompt initiation of therapy. The chemotherapeutic regimens employed in patients with highly aggressive lymphoma comprise high-dose methotrexate, which is highly teratogenic to the foetus. Hence, pregnancy termination should be strongly recommended in such cases.

Acute leukaemia

Acute leukaemia requires immediate full treatment, regardless of gestational stage.

Acute Myeloid Leukaemia

The standard induction regimen for acute myeloid leukaemia (AML) patients includes cytarabine and an anthracycline. Cytarabine, being an antimetabolite, is known to be teratogenic in animal models. The anthracycline idarubicin, is more lipophilic and therefore has an elevated placental transfer; it is also known to have higher affinity to DNA. Hence, idarubicin should be avoided during pregnancy, as it is associated with a higher prevalence of adverse foetal outcomes. The administration of induction chemotherapy during the first trimester should be preceded by a strong recommendation for pregnancy termination.

Acute Promyelocytic Leukaemia

Acute promyelocytic leukaemia induction therapy comprises all-trans-retinoic acid (ATRA) and anthracyclines. ATRA should be avoided during the first trimester due to teratogenicity.

Acute Lymphoblastic Leukaemia

Before 20th week of gestation, termination of pregnancy is recommended followed by immediate chemotherapy. After the 20th week of pregnancy, the treatment protocol, not including methotrexate, can be used before the third trimester. In the third trimester, the protocols is similar to as it is in nonpregnant patients.

Multiple Myeloma

Pregnant women diagnosed with progressive disease need immediate treatment. Steroids have proven to be the safest therapy during pregnancy, and in symptomatic myeloma patients it should be continued until delivery. In rapidly progressive disease, durig first trimester, combination therapy should be given and termination of pregnancy is to be recommended. In rapidly progressive cases later in pregnancy, chemotherapy is advisable.

Chronic Myeloid Leukaemia (CML)

As CML is a chronic disease, two scenarios may occur. The first is when a woman with CML treated with imatinib or other tyrosine kinase inhibitors wishes to become pregnant; the other is when CML is newly diagnosed during pregnancy. Imatinib exposure in pregnancy poses an increased risk for significant congenital malformations. Therefore, it should be avoided during pregnancy. Patients in the second or third trimesters who do not tolerate interferon may be treated with hydroxyurea or possibly imatinib. Leukapheresis may also be used as a transient tool for leukoreduction.

Myeloproliferative Neoplasms (MPNs)

MPN patients at a high-risk for pregnancy-related complications include women who had a prior thrombotic or haemorrhagic event; women who had pregnancy-related complications in previous pregnancies. During pregnancy, phlebotomies should be carried out, if indicated, to keep haematocrit level less than 45%. The European Leukaemia Net has published consensus-based recommendations for MPN treatment during pregnancy according to patient specific risk factors.

Blood and Blood Component Therapy

Blood products are living tissue and are used in patient care. Blood components include whole blood itself, packed red blood cells, fresh frozen plasma, cryoprecipitate, platelets, granulocyte components, and Rhogam. Because whole blood and blood components come from human blood, there is a risk of infectious disease transmission despite meticulous screening.

Blood components may contain small amounts of immunising substances and other components. Because of risks, the need for transfusion should be specific.

Historical time line

- 7th century—first recorded transfusion (from man to animal).
- 1901—Karl Landsteiner's discovery of ABO grouping laid foundation for scientific transfusion practices.
- 1920's—development of anticoagulation solutions to store donated blood.
- 1950's—disposable plastic systems for collection and aseptic separation of blood components came into use.

Ethical Aspects of Blood Donation

To ensure the safety of both donors and patients, transactions of human blood and blood components should comply with the well-acknowledged principles of biomedical ethics, namely autonomy, beneficence, nonmaleficence and justice.

Dignity also applies to donors in the sense of prohibiting the use of the human body as a source of financial gain. Respecting the rights and ensuring the safety and well-being of both donors and patients is fundamental. Consequently, blood donation should begin with a consideration of a number of ethical issues, which include:

1. Encouraging voluntary non-remunerated blood donation which serves as an important foundation for a safe and sustainable blood supply.
2. Providing information to the donor regarding the potential risks associated with the donation, the risk of donating infected blood, and the donor's responsibility with respect to patient safety and well-being.
3. Obtaining the donor's consent to the donation and to the use of the donation either for transfusion or for further manufacturing of PDMPs (plasma-derived medicinal product). The donor must be mentally competent and the consent given voluntarily. Collection of plasma for PDMPs should be undertaken only after ensuring sufficient plasma for transfusion. The use of blood and blood components for other purposes should only be allowed when self-sufficiency in blood and blood components for transfusion is already ensured. Their use in

research requires ethics approval and a separate and specific informed consent. Under national laws, exceptions may apply in situations where the donation is anonymised.

4. Encouraging "non-directed donations" (that is, donations made independently of the needs of a particular patient) in order to prevent coercion by known donors/family members, as such coercion could result in a reluctance to disclose behaviours associated with infectious risks. An exception could be made for designated donations based on medical reasons (e.g. for patients with rare blood types where no compatible non-directed donations are available).

5. Minimising the impact of deferrals on donors (e.g. health concerns, or feelings of rejection or discrimination) by educating staff on donor-deferral criteria and communication to ensure they are able to explain the reasons for deferral to donors and to follow up with deferred donors as appropriate.

6. Protecting donor health and safety during the collection of blood and blood components and, if needed, dealing with donor adverse reactions and obtaining medical care for the donor for an appropriate period of time after the collection.

7. Informing donors of abnormal test results and ensuring that reactive infectious disease test results are confirmed and the donors counselled with respect to further investigation and management by an appropriately specialised physician.

8. Protecting donors against exploitation.

9. Avoiding incentives that could influence an individual's decision to donate.

10. Protecting personal data and making them accessible only to authorised personnel such as physicians or the responsible person.

Blood Component Preparation

Blood components prepared by using either a manual or automated procedure.

The Manual Method

It involves the centrifugation of a unit of whole blood at low speed to obtain RBCs and platelet rich plasma (PRP), the transfer of the PRP into a satellite blood bag and centrifugation of the PRP at high speed to obtain the platelets and plasma. Alternatively, whole blood can be centrifuged at high speed to obtain three layers consisting of RBCs, plasma and a buffy coat containing platelets and leukocytes. The buffy coats derived from approximately 4–6 units are then pooled and centrifuged at low speed to separate the platelets from the leukocytes. The RBCs, whole blood and platelet components should be leukocyte reduced by the use of pre-storage filters.

Automated Procedure

It involves the use of apheresis machines that separate whole blood into its components, transfer the desired components into containers and return the remaining components to the donor. Some apheresis machines have built-in leukocyte-reduction mechanisms.

General principles of blood transfusion as per RCOG green Top guidelines

- Consent for blood transfusion:
  - Valid consent should be obtained where possible prior to administering a blood transfusion.

- In an emergency, where it is not feasible to get consent, information on blood transfusion should be provided retrospectively.
- The reason for transfusion and a note of the consent discussion should be documented in the patient's case notes.
- Requirements for group and screen samples and cross-matching:
  - All women should have their blood group and antibody status checked at booking and at 28 weeks of gestation.
  - Group and screen samples used for provision of blood in pregnancy should be less than 3 days old. In a woman at high-risk of emergency transfusion, e.g. placenta previa, and with no clinically significant alloantibodies, group and screen samples should be sent once a week to exclude or identify any new antibody formation and to keep blood available if necessary. Close liaison with the hospital transfusion laboratory is essential.
- Blood product specification in pregnancy and the puerperium
  - ABO, rhesus D (RhD)- and K (Kell)- compatible red cell units should be transfused. If clinically significant red cell antibodies are present, then blood negative for the relevant antigen should be cross-matched before transfusion; close liaison with the transfusion laboratory is essential to avoid delay in transfusion in life-threatening haemorrhage.
  - Cytomegalovirus (CMV)- seronegative red cell and platelet components should be provided for elective transfusions during pregnancy.

What blood components to be used!!!!

Packed red blood cell transfusion

There are no firm criteria for initiating red cell transfusion.

The decision to provide blood transfusion should be made on clinical and haematological grounds.

Indications

- Acute loss of >25% blood volume.
- Hb <8 gm/dL in perioperative period.
- Hb <8 gm/dL and symptomatic.
- Aplastic vs haemolytic anaemia.

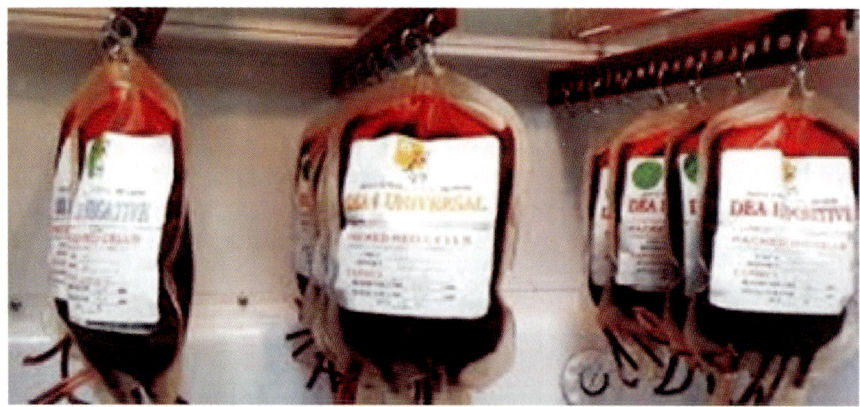

Fig. 18.1: Packed red blood cell

Packed red blood cell (Fig 18.2)

Anticoagulant—CPDA/CPD

Volume—150–200 mL

Shelf-life—21–42 days (depending on the anticoagulant)

HCT—60–80%

Storage—It must be stored in the refrigerator at 2–60°C

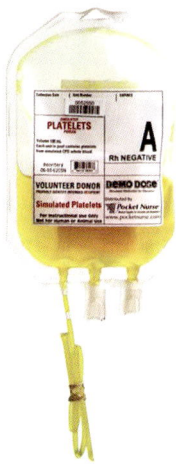

Fig. 18.2: Platelet bag

- Administration of PRBC
  - Cross matching: Compatibility; PRBCs blood must be ABO and Rh compatible with the recipient and both blood group O negative and O positive are considered to be universal blood type, can be given to patient with any other type. In an extreme situation and when the blood group is unknown, group O RhD-negative red cells should be given (although they may be incompatible for patients with irregular antibodies).
  - Catheter size->22G: Separate line for transfusion.
  - Use filter: Transfusion of whole blood and all blood components must be transfused through a filter designed to remove clots and aggregates in 0.9% sodium chloride without any other medications or solutions.
  - Method: Universal precautions to be taken during the procedure. Patient identification before transfusion to be confirmed. Blood may be warmed prior to administration for exchange or massive transfusions or for patients with cold-reactive antibodies.
- Volume-depends on indication.

Can be calculated by

The dose of whole blood is given by volume needed (mL) = (Hb desired-Hb current) × weight of the patient (kg) × 4 constant OR 20 mL/kg.

Dose of one unit compatible red blood cells will increase the haemoglobin level in an average sized adult who is not bleeding or haemolysing by approximately 1 gm/dL or Hct by 3%.

- **Infusion time:**
  The initial administration of blood is very slow should a life-threatening reaction occur.
  Within 30 minutes after removal from the refrigerator and completed within 4 hours of commencement.
  If additional transfusion are required and the time period since the last transfusion is more than 72 hours, a new sample shall be submitted to perform compatibility testing.
- **Monitor patients vital be:**
  Note patients vital parameter before transfusion and strict monitoring during and even after procedure is needed.
  Documentation of blood transfusion with indication of transfusion should be done on patient case paper.

Platelet transfusion

Aim to maintain the platelet count above $50 \times 10^9/L$ in the acutely bleeding patient. A platelet transfusion trigger of $75 \times 10^9/L$ is recommended to provide a margin of safety.

- Types:
  - Isolation from a unit of donated blood (RDP) (50–60 mL).
  - Apheresis from a single donor (SDP) (150–300 mL).
  - 1 SDP = 4–6 RDP.

  One unit of platelets is a concentrate of platelets separated from a single unit of whole blood in 40–70 mL of plasma containing 5.5×10 to the tenth power platelets
- Indications:
  - < 50000/mm³ and bleeding
  - < 50000/mm³ and invasive procedure
  - < 20000/mm³ and with risk factors
  - < 10000/mm³ without risk factors.
- Storage: Room temperature under constant agitation
- Shelf-life: 5 days
- Dose
  - 1 U RDP/10 kg body weight, or
  - 10 mL/kg (increases platelet count by 30000/mm³)

  One unit of platelets (Fig. 18.3) should increase the platelet count by 5–10,000 in a normal size .
- Administration Rate—Over 20–30 minutes.

  Crossmatch testing is not necessary when transfusing platelets. The platelets should ideally be group compatible. RhD-negative women should also receive RhD-negative platelets.

Fresh frozen plasma (FFP) (Fig. 18.3)

Plasma frozen At –18 to –300°C within 8 hours
Shelf-life—1 year
volume—200–250 mL
Ideally thawed in Blood Bank.

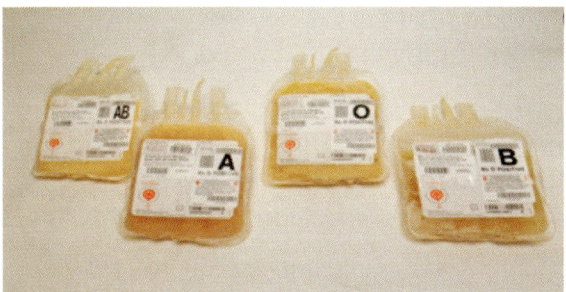

Fig. 18.3: Fresh frozen plasma

ABO matching

Donor plasma contains A and/or B alloantibodies.

Must be either ABO-identical or ABO-compatible with the recipient.

A patient with type A blood can accept plasma from donors who are type A (identical) or type AB (compatible).

A patient with type B blood can accept plasma from donors who are type B (identical) or type AB (compatible).

A patient with type O blood can accept plasma from donors who are type O (identical) or types A, B, or AB (compatible).

A patient with type AB blood can only accept plasma from donors who are type AB (identical).

If unavailable, FFP of a different ABO group is acceptable providing that it does not have a high titre of anti-A or anti-B activity. No anti-D prophylaxis is required if RhD-negative woman receives RhD-positive FFP.

Fresh frozen plasma must be ABO compatible with the recipient's red blood cells, but compatibility testing is not necessary. Fresh frozen plasma (FPP) contains all of the coagulation factors.

- Indications
  - Congenital single factor deficiency, e.g. haemophilia (if no factor concentrate available) and hereditary clotting factor deficiencies like von Willebrand disease.
  - Vitamin K deficiency associated with active bleeding.
  - Used in treatment of haemorrhagic disease of the newborn; use FFP and intravenous vitamin.
  - Reversal of warfarin if the patient is bleeding.
  - Thrombotic thrombocytopenic purpura (TTP) or haemolytic uremic syndrome (HUS).
  - Replacement of multiple clotting factor deficiencies in bleeding patients who have significant coagulopathy (defined as PT>18 sec, or PTT>55 sec) due to multiple factor deficiencies, e.g. massive transfusion, DIC, vitamin K deficiency.
- Dose—10 mL/kg

In massive blood loss and blood component replacement, one unit of FFP is transfused for each two to three units of packed red blood cells. Subsequent FFP transfusion should be guided by the results of clotting tests if they are available in a timely manner, aiming to maintain prothrombin time (PT) and activated partial thromboplastin time (APTT) ratios at less than 1.5 × normal.

It is essential that regular full blood counts and coagulation screens (PT, APTT and fibrinogen) are performed during the bleeding episode.

Cryoprecipitate (Fig. 18.4)

When cryoprecipitate is administered, ABO compatibility is preferred without consideration of Rh status. Compatibility testing is unnecessary. No anti-D prophylaxis is required if a RhD-negative woman receives RhD-positive cryoprecipitate.

The cryoprecipitate is mixed well with 10–15 mL of 0.9% sodium chloride.

- Preparation—Plasma is frozen for 24 hours, and then thawed at 1–6°C until insoluble proteins precipitate. The pack is centrifuged to obtain the cryoprecipitate. The cryoprecipitate is then refrozen for storage.

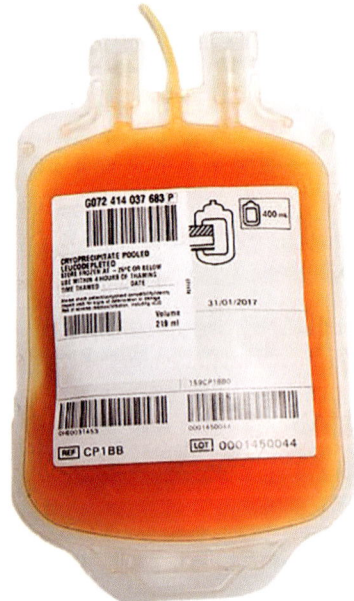

Fig. 18.4: Cryoprecipitate

Contains

FVIII: C, von Willebrand factor (vWF), fibrinogen, FXIII, and fibronectin.

Cryoprecipitate has the following factor activities

91 IU of FVIII: C per bag,

113 IU of vWF per bag,

150 mg of fibrinogen per bag

Once thawed, the product should be transfused immediately, with completion of transfusion within 4 hours of issuing product.

- Indications:
  - *von* Willebrand disease
  - Haemophilia A

- Factor XIII deficiency
- DIC
- Dys and hypofibrinogenemia

Dose—One Unit per 7–10 kg BW.

number of bags of cryoprecipitate =

[(plasma volume in mL % increase in F VIII: C needed)/100]/80

Risks of Blood and Blood Components

Blood transfusion carries the risk of transmitting infections if the donated blood contains pathogens.

As the collection of blood requires a venepuncture to be performed, pathogenic bacteria could be transferred into the donation from a contaminated skin area and subsequently proliferate (particularly in platelets) to clinically significant numbers capable of causing an RTTI, i.e. relevant transfusion-transmitted infection(s). This risk must be minimised by the use of standardised and validated techniques and disinfectants for aseptic venepuncture. Moreover, thorough adherence to aseptic technique with closed systems and appropriate microbiological sterility testing should be implemented.

In the case of several pathogens causing severe disease (including HIV, HBV and HCV) an exposed donor harbouring an RTTI may feel well and wish to donate despite being at risk of transmitting infections to patients. Therefore, it is crucial to:

a. Collect blood from voluntary non-remunerated donors, as they are known to have lower rates of RTTI.

b. Exclude from donating, through enquiry, any person who has been at increased risk of acquiring such an infection.

c. Test all donors for RTTI using validated assays that have been approved by relevant regulatory authorities.

Donors who have tested positive on a first or previous donation must be systematically deferred, i.e. the donation must not enter the processing and testing cycle. To achieve this it is recommended that:

a. A national blood donor registry (e.g. as part of the blood management system) is maintained at all points of donation.

b. Donors are registered using a unique-identifier system. Conditions for the potential re-entry of donors (e.g. after proven clearance of the infection or demonstration of a false-positive test) may be defined.

There are also a number of adverse reactions due to immunological mechanisms; the most relevant of these is blood group incompatibility. Therefore, careful blood group typing and documentation is essential to avoid errors (e.g. giving the wrong blood to the patient).

The risks associated with blood transfusion necessitate traceability from donor to patient and vice versa, and a system of haemovigilance, i.e. documenting and reporting adverse events and reactions, and initiating corrective actions where necessary. The management of risks associated with blood transfusion needs to be part of the quality management system developed by the blood establishment.

Suggested Reading

1. Principles and practice in immunohematology second edition by Eva D. Quinley.
2. Guide to the preparation, use and quality assurance of blood components (European countries).
3. Green-top guideline no. 47 May 2015 'Blood transfusion in obstetrics'.
4. BC medical journal volume 49 no. 8, October 2007 'Guidelines for cryoprecipitate transfusion'.
5. Williams Obstetrics 24th edition 'Haematological disorders in pregnancy'.
6. High-risk pregnancy management option volume (1) 5th edition 'Anaemia in white blood cells in pregnancy'.
7. WHO manual of blood transfusion.
8. Wintrobe's Haematology 'Anaemia'.

Index